Many times during my pregnancy I found myself wishing that I had a friend who'd already had twins who could share her experiences with me, who could calm my fears, alert me to what might come next, and laugh with me over the astounding proportions of my belly. . . . That's the final reason this book came to be. I hope it will be just that kind of helpful companion for you as you undertake the incredible journey that is a twin pregnancy.

—JANE SEYMOUR,
from her prologue in

Two at a Time

With the warm and reas_____ been there, Jane Seymour explains the spe_____, _____lenges that are unique to twin pregnancy—and offers sound advice on:

- why twin pregnancies are usually shorter in length than single-child pregnancies

- why almost everyone who is pregnant with twins becomes anemic

- how the nesting instinct kicks in to an even greater effect when you're pregnant with twins

- why some twins tend to develop apnea

- how to maintain a healthy exercise regimen when you're eating for three . . . and much more!

Two at a Time

Having Twins: The Journey Through Pregnancy and Birth

Jane Seymour
and
Pamela Patrick Novotny

With a Foreword by Sheryl Ross, M.D.

A FIRESIDE BOOK
Published by Simon & Schuster
New York London Toronto Sydney Singapore

The authors of this book are not physicians, and the ideas, procedures, and suggestions in this book are not intended as a substitute for the medical advice of a trained health professional. All matters regarding your health require medical supervision. Consult your physician before adopting the suggestions in this book, as well as about any condition that may require diagnosis or medical attention. The authors and publisher disclaim any liability arising directly or indirectly from the use of this book.

 FIRESIDE
Rockefeller Center
1230 Avenue of the Americas
New York, NY 10020

First Fireside Edition 2002
FIRESIDE and colophon are registered trademarks
of Simon & Schuster, Inc.

For information about special discounts for bulk purchases,
please contact Simon & Schuster Special Sales at
1-800-456-6798 or business@simonandschuster.com

Designed by Nancy Singer

Manufactured in the United States of America

10 9 8 7 6 5 4 3 2 1

ISBN 0-671-03677-7
    0-671-03678-5 (Pbk)

*I dedicate this book to James, my wonderful husband
whose inspiration, patience, and compassion allowed
our miracle to come true. And of course John and Kris
who inspire us daily; and to our doctors Sheryl Ross and
Rick Paulson who made it all possible.*

❧

*To Jerry especially, for his heart and his mind.
He and Anna, Claire, Rachel, Sam and Eli, have shown
me how loving, fulfilling and fun families can be.*

Acknowledgments

When people share their knowledge wholeheartedly, the result can't help but be wonderful. That's what happened with this book, and those who contributed what they know are owed a sincere vote of thanks. My thanks go to Dr. Lisa Stern, and especially Dr. Sheryl Ross who spent many hours sharing medical details. Thanks must also go to Cheri Ingle, Andrea Daoutis and Sarah Bishop, all of whom helped make my job not only easy, but enjoyable.

Foreword

I have known Jane and James for nearly ten years. We started as doctor and patient, but over the years, we have become friends. Because of our friendship, I was happy to be with them—physically as well as emotionally—during their long journey from fertility treatments through the difficult pregnancy Jane experienced before they held their sons, Kristopher and John, in their arms.

Like so many women today who delay childbearing until they are in their late 30s or 40s, Jane wanted this pregnancy badly. Many women in this age group are attempting their first pregnancy, but for Jane and James, finding each other after previous marriages strengthened their desire for a baby, even though they knew how difficult it would be. Fortunately, they were able to use the wonderful developments in fertility treatments to achieve their desire. Still, theirs was a confusing, frustrating and difficult road.

In so many ways, their experience is similar to that of many thousands of couples in this country. The key to finally achieving their pregnancy was that they remained hopeful, even after Jane's miscarriages. In a similar way, I encourage my patients who are still trying to get pregnant using fertility treatments to have faith that they'll find a treatment that works for them. There are so many alternatives now, and it just takes time to find the right one.

When that pregnancy finally happens, and the couple finds out they have twins, that news really can double the joy, as it did for Jane and James. But it can also pose special risks to the mother and to her babies, particularly if the mother is over 40. Medical textbooks list common complications in twin pregnancies for women in this age group: premature labor, premature rupture of membranes, maternal high blood pressure and preeclampsia, gestational diabetes and intrauterine growth retardation of the babies. And Jane was a textbook case. She took great care of herself during her pregnancy, but just as the medical textbooks predict, because of her age she developed preeclampsia. The good news is that through early detection and continued care, she nevertheless had a good outcome: two healthy babies.

In order to lower your risk of complications, I urge you to take care of the basics: eat well, gain 35 to 45 pounds during your pregnancy, get adequate rest, and exercise reasonably during and after your pregnancy.

To be certain it's clear exactly how to do all that, I recommend a team approach. Seeing a nutritionist during the early stages of your pregnancy can help you set up a healthful diet for you and your babies. You could also talk with your doctor about seeing a perinatalogist, an obstetrical consultant specially trained in handling high-risk pregnancies. And, a person specifically trained in safe exercise methods for pregnancy can also be a big help. The more supportive and comprehensive your team is, the more likely it is that your pregnancy will be successful and free of complications.

Your commitment to this pregnancy and this process, like the commitment that Jane and James made to theirs, is the best insurance you can provide for your babies.

Dr. Sheryl Ross
Santa Monica, California
June 2000

Contents

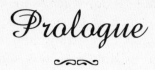

Prologue

One baby is a miracle. To be given two at once is a gift beyond words. Like you, my husband and I longed for a baby, and we were delighted but a bit overwhelmed when we found that not one, but two were on the way. Our fraternal boys, Kristopher and John, are school age already; their early years have absolutely sped by. But we continue to feel so grateful for them, and are continually amazed by them in so many ways. We love to compare notes with other parents of twins like you and to share what we have learned. And that's partly why this book was born.

I suppose you could say that it really had its beginnings when James and I met. I had just finished shooting the pilot for *Dr. Quinn, Medicine Woman* and of course had no idea if it would be picked up as a series. In the meantime, I was producing my first movie and I needed a director and co-producer with plenty of experience. After a bit of a search my agent announced, "I've found the perfect person for the job, and it's someone you're going to love—James Keach!" Little did any of us know how prophetic those words would turn out to be.

From the moment I sat down across the table from him at the restaurant where we met, it seemed James could see straight through me to whatever I was truly thinking or feeling. As we worked on the project, I found he was someone I could really communicate with at a level I'd never experienced. It was surprising because most men don't easily speak on emotional or spiritual terms as James does. Soon enough we realized that working together was going to be fabulous, exciting, and that neither of us wanted our time together to end once the film project was over.

I was 43 when we married. We both knew from the beginning that we wanted to have a baby together, even though we both had children from previous marriages. There are a million reasons why any couple wants to have children, and I daresay that for each couple those reasons are a unique and intimate part of their relationship. Part of it for us was that we both had been through so much before we met, and we wanted to start over, to make our families new again with each other. A baby we had together would be a sign of a new beginning for us, and that was important. But even more than that, I felt strongly that I wanted another child, and I wanted that child with James. In loving me and in being so immediately sensitive to me, James had already given me so much. More than anything I longed to give him something wonderful in return that no one else could offer. I wanted to give James a baby and a happy family life.

We started right away trying to have a baby, and because of my age and the rather impatient nature James and I share, we asked for help early on. Mercifully, the options available to couples who want a baby are extraordinary. James and I immediately committed to doing everything we could to have a baby, and promised each other that we'd face this uphill struggle together.

And struggle we did. If you've been through infertility treatment, as so many parents of twins have, you know the hopes and disappointments are *huge*. Somehow you look around and everyone else seems to be getting pregnant without even trying. There you are, getting injections, taking pills. I was an emotional mess during that time; so much up-and-down, up-and-down. I'd simply become another person because of the injections, especially the Pergonal. We used to call it Pergonal Hell. The doctor had said, "Well, you might have some mood swings as a result of the injections." Mood swings! These were not gentle shifts. These were wild, maniacal episodes. I'm usually relatively sane, but I had some feelings and emotional responses because of the drugs, that I don't know *where* they came from.

As he'd promised he would be, James was a great support. No matter how nasty or irrational I was, he'd just hold me, and I'd cry and cry and cry. In the middle of it all I thought, "What an enormous test this is. You'd have to want a baby desperately to stay with this madness!"

We, like many of you, did want that baby desperately, and as soon as we found out we were having twins, we were both deliriously happy, on top of the world. It felt like we'd not only passed the test, but that we'd earned an A-plus! But our pregnancy "honeymoon" didn't last long. In spite of that A-plus, I quickly found I had a lot to learn, beginning with the idea that even though *getting* pregnant seemed a huge triumph, *being* pregnant with twins presented a whole new set of challenges. It didn't matter that I'd been pregnant with one baby twice before; this was different. The first time I had to carry a wastebasket for vomiting with me from my makeup trailer to the set of *Dr. Quinn,* (my stomach was *that* unsettled) it really sank in how very different this pregnancy was going to be. Looking back, I almost cringe when I recall how blithely I had assured Beth Sullivan, the creator and producer of *Dr. Quinn,* that my pregnancy, even though it was a twin pregnancy, wouldn't affect our shooting schedule for the show. I made good on my assurances, but you'll understand when I tell you there were times when it required monumental effort to do so.

And that's another reason this book came to be. As it turned out, I did play the part of a pioneer doctor on television for years, and I'm keenly interested in homeopathic care and other forms of alternative medicine. My acting experience made me comfortable with a certain amount of medical information, but once I was pregnant with twins, I was in unexplored territory, and I was driven to find out more. I turned to every book I could lay my hands on to get the information I needed. I wanted to know in detail what I could expect during this pregnancy. I wanted to know what was happening to me, how my babies were growing, what I could do to have the healthiest pregnancy possible, and how to prepare for the ups and downs peculiar to twin pregnancy I might need to be prepared for. I looked first to books to find answers to my questions, just as you are looking to this book to be your companion throughout your twin pregnancy.

In these pages I share what I found out from my own doctor, pediatrician, alternative health practitioners and many of the top experts in the fields of twin pregnancy, nutrition, and neonatology. And I'm happy to share, too, what I learned firsthand: that sometimes twin pregnancy can be relatively uneventful with the mom working, running errands and chasing her other kids around. But I also learned that it can change overnight, landing mom on bed rest, worrying about her unborn babies, wondering how to keep her sanity, and trying to figure out how to run a household from her bedside. It's all here for you, presented a trimester at a time along with information and tips on preparing for the first months after your babies are born.

Many times during my pregnancy I found myself wishing that I had a friend who'd already had twins who could share her experiences with me, who could calm my fears, alert me to what might come next, and laugh with me over the astounding proportions of my belly without thinking I was odd, or making silly comments that showed she didn't understand what it was like to occupy such a rapidly expanding body.

That's the final reason this book came to be. I hope it will be just that kind of helpful companion for you as you undertake the incredible journey that is a twin pregnancy.

one

Precious Cargo

ow did you find out you were carrying the most precious cargo of all? Many women I've talked to tell me they knew they were pregnant before a test confirmed it for them. Some just had a sort of sixth sense about it, others felt too edgy to believe they were simply premenstrual. One friend was certain she was coming down with the flu, she was so tired, until she realized she'd been "coming down with something" for weeks, and the "something" had never materialized—but neither had her period!

With my other pregnancies, there were always two infallible early signs: suddenly, strong smells were upsetting to me; I couldn't even bear the scent of my favorite perfume. But most of all, I was tired, a word that's not usually part of my vocabulary. Those symptoms always set me to wondering enough to go to the doctor for a pregnancy test.

When I got pregnant with our twins, because we were assisted by technology and I was closely monitored, I hardly had a moment to wonder what was happening. Before I had time to develop symptoms to wonder about, I knew not only that I was pregnant, but that it would be twins. I'd stepped immediately into a phase unique to women like you and me—that of wondering about how and why these two embryos, these twins, came to grow inside of us.

One Egg, or Two?

My boys have a strong family resemblance to each other, but they are fraternal. Still, people are forever asking me if they are identical. More to the point, they also ask me how I can be *sure* whether they're

What's the Difference Between Fraternal and Identical Twins?

Twins come in two forms: identical, which are formed from a single egg fertilized by a single sperm which splits to form two babies; and fraternal, which are formed when two separate eggs are fertilized by two sperm and each implants in the womb. The majority of twins, about two-thirds, are fraternal.

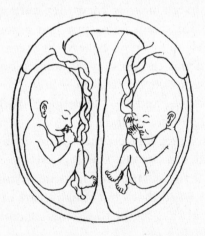

Two sacs with one fused placenta.

identical or fraternal. Usually, I simply smile and tell them to look a little more carefully at the boys, and they'll see the differences.

With closer friends I tell them I know because all babies conceived with help, as ours were, are fraternal. Fertility treatments—in all the forms that have to do with women's reproductive systems—simply encourage the ovaries to produce more eggs, not to make them split. And if you've been through fertility treatments, I don't have to tell you the details of how they work. When James and I were going through that process, we ended up feeling that

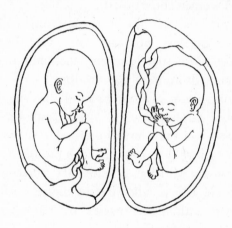

Two sacs with two placentas.

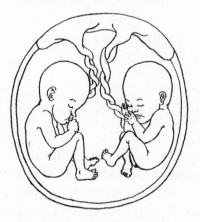

One sac with one placenta.

Who Has Fraternal Twins?

You're more likely to have fraternal twins if you are:

- Black. We don't know exactly why, but presumably black women all over the world are more likely to release more than one egg each month than women of other races. Overall, black women hold the title for the highest rate of fraternal twinning, Caucasian women are in second place, and Asian women come in last.
- In your 30s. See above: some women in their 30s, regardless of race, are more likely to release more than one egg each month. That tendency disappears in your 40s.
- A woman whose *mother's* family seems to have a lot of *fraternal* twins. Again, same reason as above—you may have inherited a tendency to release more than one egg each month.
- A woman who has already had three or four children. This is called having higher parity, and women with higher parity are more likely to have fraternal twins.
- A woman who got pregnant within a month of stopping birth control pills. There seems to be a rebound effect for some women, causing the release of more than one egg.

we knew far more than we had ever dreamed we'd know (or honestly, *wanted* to know!) about conception. Suffice it to say that, no matter how they were produced, when two fertilized eggs implant in the uterus, you're having fraternal twins.

Identical twins are another matter altogether. Because they come from a single fertilized egg, identical twins have identical

DNA, and of course, unlike my boys, they really do look alike. If your twins were conceived without medical help, "the old-fashioned way," you'll not likely be able to tell whether they are identical or fraternal unless you have amniocentesis (more on such tests in Chapters 2 through 4). Ultrasound sometimes offers clues, but not always.

If you're lucky, when your babies are born, the routine examination of the placenta will show that your babies had one of everything—one inner sac, one outer sac and one placenta—then you'll know they are identical. Any other combination for babies conceived without help means the decision, fraternal or identical, is up for further analysis.

You can have DNA tests done on your babies, but they are very expensive, and most doctors will tell you they're not worth it unless there's some medical problem you're trying to sort out. Or, you can simply wait and see how they look!

Are There More Twins Being Born Today?

If it seems you're seeing twins everywhere, you are. Twins happen much more frequently than they used to. Just a few years ago twins showed up once in about every 80-90 births; now it's once in 41 births in the U.S.!

First Feelings

Immediately on the heels of the wild, incredible, unbelievable joy James and I felt on finding out we were pregnant, came fear. I was terrified I'd lose these babies as I'd lost two other pregnancies during our fertility treatments. One miscarriage had occurred very early on in the pregnancy, and was not much more than a heavy period when I knew I shouldn't be having one. The second was much more traumatic and frightening. It happened while I was on live national television, co-hosting the New Year's Day parade in New York. By the time I felt the cramping, it was too late. The moment we were off the air, James carried me to a nearby hospital where the doctor confirmed that I had miscarried. We were brokenhearted.

So this time, when I was told I was pregnant, I was afraid to move. Swing dancing was out—and James and I had fallen in love dancing, so even though it may sound unimportant, it was a kind of loss for us, but certainly one we could live with. At work on the set of *Dr. Quinn,* we made some alterations immediately. I could sit on a horse or in a wagon, but I wasn't going to jump up onto either of those, even though the story line routinely called for me to do that. So we got a body double for me, and she did the leaping, the jumping and the sliding into home plate as one episode required soon after my positive pregnancy test. I was happy and relieved we could do that, but it made me think of how hard it is for women who are not actresses, who never get a body double for hard work they have to do in normal life, difficult pregnancy or no. Wouldn't it be great if we could all have a body double to stand in for us when we're feeling especially fragile—or when we actually *are* especially fragile?

I have to admit that feeling so afraid and vulnerable early in my pregnancy was disconcerting. Perhaps you've felt that kind of fear and worry, too. I hope it will be comforting for you to know that for me—and I think for many women—the fear did pass, especially as I worked hard to do all I could to take care of myself and of my babies, and as I learned more about what was happening to me, and to them. And I tried to be philosophical. I'd psyche myself up by telling myself "I will do all I can to achieve my goal," and then in my mind I sort of let go of the end result, even while I'm trying my best to make sure it has every chance of happening. That's what I did early on in my twin pregnancy. I focused on what I *could do* rather than dwelling on what frightened me or on what I could not control.

I also tried to laugh as much as possible. It seemed to lighten the dire atmosphere I could so easily create for myself. Out of necessity, James and I began to find humor in some pretty strange situations. If you've had difficulty keeping a pregnancy, or if you've undergone fertility treatments, you'll be familiar with the progesterone injections (or suppositories) necessary to be sure the embryos implant in the wall of the uterus and stay there until the placenta (or placentas) can begin making enough progesterone on its *(their)* own. By that time I'd had so many injections, James and I often joked about feeling like junkies—always looking for a private place to "shoot up." I remember going to a certain glamorous black-tie Hollywood event and in my tiny jeweled evening bag I carried, not just a lipstick, but the syringe and medication I'd need to have that evening to remain on schedule. James had to "administer" the medication because it had to go in my backside, which I couldn't reach while I was wearing my elaborate gown. But where should we go for our needle party? I couldn't go into the men's room with him, and he couldn't go into the ladies' room with me. So we roamed the corridors of this fancy hotel, looking for a deserted corner. We finally found a small, out-of-the-way alcove. Crowding ourselves against the back wall, looking to the left, right and center, I lifted up the skirt of my huge ball gown and bent over. James, elegant in his tux, swabbed a spot on my backside with alcohol, quickly jammed in the needle, and squeezed out the medication. After I'd rearranged my dress, we walked out all smiles, as if nothing unusual had happened, although we did giggle to think of how many other couples were doing something similar, perhaps not in ball gown and tux, but definitely involving needles at inconvenient times.

Of course not all twin pregnancies are so delicate. By now you may have heard that about half of all twins are born early. That means, happily, that the other half are born at full term, which for twins is 36–38 weeks. Many women have complications in twin pregnancies, but just as many do not. You may be like a friend of mine who didn't even find out she was having twins until she was 28 weeks pregnant! She'd been blithely attending her ballet classes right up until the ultrasound that showed two babies occupying her previously unexplainably large belly. And there are still a few delivery-table surprises—births where the "placenta" turns out to be a second baby. The key to a healthy pregnancy, I believe, is to keep close track of what's happening in your pregnancy by having good prenatal care, eating well, and exercising appropriately. Keep yourself healthy, and you can be ready for what your pregnancy brings you.

The "Older Mother" Myth

If there's one thing I learned very early in my pregnancy, it's that there is a kind of myth or misunderstanding about those of us who are considered "older" mothers. I was 45 when our boys were born, and I have to admit that I had some questions about how my age would affect my babies. I'd heard somewhere—who knows where—that pregnancy was somehow perilous for women of my age. James and I had worked so hard to *get* pregnant, I hadn't really stopped to think about whether the pregnancy itself would be any more difficult for me because of my age than it would be if I were younger.

After the first few comments from well-meaning friends about my age and their concerns for my pregnancy, I went looking for more information. Here's the good news I found—the most recent thinking in much of the medical community is that in a sense, the risk associated with older mothers and their pregnancies has often been overstated. The fact is that if a woman is healthy and fit, her uterus is likely also to be healthy and fit. It's true that older eggs can mean a higher risk of genetic problems, but screening techniques continue to help in that area. And careful monitoring makes a difference, too. Women over 40 are at higher risk for hypertension, preeclampsia and gestational diabetes, but as I found out in my own pregnancy, thankfully there are many ways to monitor for and treat these conditions.

All this made a lot of sense to me. I think women in their 30s and 40s are far more responsible in lots of ways than they were when they were in their 20s. I *know* I am! All those years of life experience and the emotional preparation and planning that can go into getting pregnant can actually help older women have healthier pregnancies. I know my body and what it needs better now than ever before, and if you are an "older mother," too, I'm sure you feel that way as well. So when it comes to choosing healthy behaviors or fine-tuning your lifestyle for the sake of your babies, an older mom often knows just what to do. If she doesn't, you can bet she will find out, and do it!

That, of course, is not to say that younger moms are irresponsible. Youth, not to speak of stomach muscles that haven't been stretched to the limit by previous babies, are definite pluses where pregnancy is concerned! At the end of the day, whether you count yourself as a younger mom or an older mom, I believe it's the wisdom you bring to your pregnancy and the willingness to make healthy decisions for yourself and your babies that make all the difference.

Who *Are* You Going to Call?

Even though I was being closely monitored during our efforts to get pregnant, James and I had a home pregnancy test kit ready and waiting for the right moment. Haven't these simple little kits made an enormous difference for us? With my earlier pregnancies, I remember waiting until my doctor's office called to confirm my suspicions so that I could say that I was officially pregnant. Now it's often reversed: the woman calls the doctor to announce her pregnancy, and to make an appointment for her first prenatal visit. What a switch!

I have to admit that in our case, there was no romantic, candle-lit dinner, no handholding stroll along the beach near our home at sunset, no intimate tête-à-tête during which I quietly announced my long-awaited pregnancy to James. The spot we most likely first shared the news that I was pregnant was in our bathroom, over the home pregnancy test which we did on our own to confirm what we thought had happened. Not much romance to it, but quite a lot of excitement. I don't actually remember the details but I know we called the doctor immediately and went directly to his office.

It's funny how, when you're trying to get pregnant, you think you'll never forget all that you went through, or the moment you finally got that positive test result. Or, if you haven't had to try so hard for babies, how easy it is to think you'll never forget the moment you got the news you were pregnant, or the moment you told your husband. I've been surprised to find that so much is eclipsed by the enormous miracle of a twin pregnancy and the birth of those babies, that sometimes it seems all that came before their birth melts into a single entity, a single piece of time. I've thought more than once that there ought to be a special name for that time in the lives of parents of twins called BB—Before Babies.

Strange as it may sound now, I never really considered ahead of time that we'd have twins, although of course I knew it was a possibility. With all the testing associated with my pregnancy, we found out right away—we knew that more than one embryo had implanted. In fact, three had implanted; the doctor showed us on the ultrasound. We could see all three clearly, and we could also see that one embryo was a quarter of the size of the other two. My doctor explained that he didn't think that embryo would develop, and that it wasn't unusual for that to happen, even in non-assisted pregnancies. Sure enough, within a week or two after we saw the three embryos on my ultrasound, the smallest of them disappeared as if by magic. It had simply been re-absorbed by my body. That process, my doctor explained, is called *vanishing twin syndrome*—or maybe in my case it should be called *vanishing triplet syndrome*. Sometimes the embryo vanishes farther into the first trimester, and then there may be some cramping or maybe even some bleeding or tissue that's passed, just as there is in a miscarriage. In those cases, the pregnancy for the remaining twin most often carries on normally. In fact, my doctor said there are probably many more twins conceived than delivered. Because we can perform early ultrasounds, for the first time ever, we can know about some of those vanishing twins, or triplets, as the case may be.

So if you've just been given the greatest news on earth—not only that you are pregnant, but that you get two babies—do you shout it from the rooftops? Do you keep it under your hat for a while? Who *do* you call? How do you decide who shares the news of the gift you've been given? That can be a tough question. In my first two pregnancies with Katie and Sean, I told just about everyone I knew right away. After letting my husband in on the news I was on the phone with my closest girlfriends, with my parents, with my sisters, and I chatted casually about my pregnancy with co-workers. With my twins though, I found that I felt a bit more circumspect.

After losing two pregnancies, fear made me more than willing to wait a while to publicly announce the fact of the third pregnancy to the world at large. Each time, many people I worked with knew I was pregnant almost as soon as I did, because they were so aware we were trying and I was updating everyone on the set. And each time, it was particularly painful to return to the set and announce I wasn't pregnant any longer. I really didn't want to go through any of that again.

As I sorted out how to deal with news of this pregnancy, I remembered a conversation I'd had with a friend that helped guide me, and perhaps it will be helpful to you too. My friend and I had talked about the difference between *private* and *secret,* and that helped me define my own boundaries concerning who would know about the pregnancy and how much they would know. My pregnancy certainly wasn't a secret, it couldn't be even if I'd wanted that. After all, nearly 200 people on the set knew within days that I'd had a positive pregnancy test because suddenly I had to have a body double. And it would only have added to the stress of the time to try to keep secret something as momentous as this pregnancy. In fact, I did feel comfortable letting those I worked with—the "family" with whom I spent 12-hour days on the set—know about the day-to-day facts of the pregnancy.

Still, there was a part of me that felt that my pregnancy was also an important, intimate and very private part of my relationship with James. That deeper part of the pregnancy I did not share with the world. I held close to my heart doubts and fears that troubled me from time to time as well as the keen sense of contentment and commitment I felt. As I let the idea of the difference between private and secret settle in my mind, I found that I was no longer dithering and afraid about who to tell and who not to tell. No matter how many people knew that I was pregnant, the deepest meanings of the pregnancy could remain private. They belonged to James and me.

two

Steps in the Journey

Weeks 4-16

When I became pregnant with our boys, I thought I knew all about pregnancy and what it would be like. After all, I'd been pregnant twice before. With both Katie and Sean I'd had delightfully uneventful pregnancies with all the usual bodily changes. I would have some queasiness from time to time during the first few months. There would be a little bump growing where my flat tummy used to be which didn't require maternity clothing until I was about six months along. And of course there were the larger breasts, which I thought were quite decorative!

So I came to my twin pregnancy thinking that of course this one would be different in some ways—I *was* having two babies after all—but that having been pregnant before, I knew what to expect.

Was I surprised! Trust me: Having twins does not mean only that your belly will get bigger than it does with one baby. That's certainly true, but I also felt that every step of the way my twin pregnancy was a totally different experience than I'd had during my other pregnancies, from how I felt, to how I looked, to what I needed to do to take care of myself. For the most part, (except for certain unpleasant aspects of the first three months) I enjoyed my pregnancy, and best of all, I had a constant sense of awe about what was taking place inside my body. I did often wish though, that there had been someone to take me aside at the start and prepare me for the intensity of the journey I was beginning!

Your Pregnant Body

First things first. I have to tell you that I was definitely not prepared for how much I threw up during the first three months. Yes, I had felt some nausea with the other pregnancies, but projectile vomiting? Never. I'm not someone who normally throws up at all, but during this pregnancy, my stomach gave me no choice. The morning sickness (which on some days would be more aptly called morning-noon-and-sometimes-night sickness) started almost immediately after I found out I was pregnant.

What Causes Morning Sickness?

Nausea that often comes with pregnancy can happen any time of the day, not just morning. There are several theories about it, but most agree that a natural increase in progesterone levels is the culprit—and when you're having twins, you get double the amount of progesterone.

My schedule on *Dr. Quinn, Medicine Woman* was quite demanding already, without figuring in time to be sick. On a typical weekday, I'd get up at 4:30 or 5:00 A.M. and first thing, I'd throw up. Then I'd shower and dress in something comfortable and loose-fitting that didn't have to be taken off over my head—perhaps a soft flannel shirt and jeans. Thank goodness I didn't have to do my own hair or makeup, and that no one would see me in what I wore to work.

Paramount Ranch, where we filmed *Dr. Quinn,* was about 15 minutes from my house, so I'd leave home at about 5:30 A.M. in order to be on the set at the required 5:45 A.M. I had this beautiful trailer which was my home base on the set, and every morning I'd walk in the door and throw up. Sometimes twice. I kept several plastic buckets in the trailer, one right by the front door, because I confess I didn't always manage to get to the bathroom. Then I would take a clean bucket and go to the makeup trailer and I'd lose it again. Poor Kelly, my hairdresser, and Lesa, my makeup artist. They had to watch me be sick every day for months!

Finding food that would stay down was a challenge. Before I was pregnant, I'd eat breakfast while Kelly and Lesa were doing my hair and makeup, but during the months I was so sick, there wasn't much breakfast I could eat. Sometimes I could get some fruit or crackers to stay down, but I did most of my eating later in the day because the nausea was at its worst in the morning. I'd still feel nauseous other times in the day, but I wouldn't necessarily lose it.

Patrice Harper, bless her, was the woman on the set who got snacks for us. She'd had children, so she knew what I was going through, and she was persistent about coming up with foods I might be able to keep down. She was the one who hit on matzoh ball soup. She would go to a nearby restaurant and pick it up. By midmorning I'd be able to just down it, a whole bowl of delicious broth with big chunks of chicken in it.

Even with my nausea, I knew that with two babies growing inside me, it was important that I find a way to eat *something.* In addition to feeling sick all the time, I was constantly putting pressure on myself to try to eat things I just couldn't stomach because I thought I ought to, then feeling defeated when I threw up and knew I had to start trying to eat all over again. Finally, seeing my predicament, my doctor said that while I was so sick, eating anything was better than nothing, and that I should eat only what appealed to me. I could improve the nutritional value of my diet and the amount I ate the moment my stomach settled down. What a relief that was! So until my stomach did settle, I decided my mantra would be *Eat Only What You Can*.

Once I felt all right about that, I turned my attention to easing the nausea. There is quite a bit of information available about what works to combat nausea for different women, but here are a few tips I found that helped me:

- I tried to keep my blood sugar on an even keel. Often a little fruit in the morning would make me feel better—it raised my blood sugar quickly. Later, I learned my blood sugar would have stayed up longer if I'd eaten some protein with the fruit. You can help raise your blood sugar quickly in the morning if you keep crackers by your bed and eat them *before* you get up. I've heard of women who would actually get up in the middle of the night to eat a bowl of cereal so that their blood sugar wouldn't drop so far by morning. That didn't sound appealing to me, but if you're desperate for a nausea-free morning, it can't hurt to try!

- I snacked frequently during the day for the same reason—to keep my blood sugar up and the nausea away. For me, the best snack was that matzoh ball soup. I also ate a lot of cracker-type snacks such as saltines, wheat thins, pretzels. I loved licorice—that was my sweet, and fortunately, natural licorice drops can be soothing to an upset stomach. Try whatever sounds appealing to you: peanut butter crackers or a sweet fruit, or a non-acidic fruit juice.

- I ate when I could. Evenings were so much easier for me. I usually didn't have trouble eating a nutritious dinner with lots of protein, say grilled fish or chicken, a salad and some potatoes, rice or bread with milk to drink, maybe frozen yogurt for dessert. I wasn't always particularly hungry at that time of day, but when I wasn't nauseous, I knew it was my one chance of the day to eat more nutritious foods, and the larger amounts, my babies needed.

What Else Can I Do for Nausea?

In twin pregnancies, nausea can last as long as 16 weeks, or even longer for some people, so it's a good idea to find some safe remedies that are helpful to you. Try peppermint or chamomile tea, B-complex vitamins, or ginger tea with a little brown sugar in it. Also worth a try are anti-nausea wristbands sold in some pharmacies and health food stores, which use an acupressure point to ease nausea.

Simply eating enough was a major issue for me during the first trimester, and I have to admit, not always a pleasant one. But I hope you'll keep in mind that for as many women who are like me, fighting to keep weight on and food down during the early months, there are just as many for whom nausea is only an occasional problem—or even non-existent. It's common to feel ravenously hungry right away, which I'm sure is your body's way of letting you know it is time to store up some extra calories for the babies. In fact, my doctor told me I should put on as much of the weight I needed to gain for the babies as early in my pregnancy as possible, that is, as soon as the nausea let up. Her reasoning was that so much of the growth and development of the babies happens early on, and that later in the pregnancy it becomes difficult to fit much food at one time in a stomach that's crowded by babies. Besides, twin pregnancies usually last closer to 36 to 38 weeks than the typical 40 weeks, so you're likely to be about a month short of weight-gaining time.

When my stomach finally sorted itself out late in the first trimester (be assured, there was an end to the nausea), I could once again eat without fear of throwing up and having to start all over again. But then I was faced with the next problem we all have to deal with when we're pregnant with twins: our culture doesn't look kindly on weight gain, does it? Most of us have trained ourselves since adolescence to avoid weight gain at all

---

How Much Weight Should I Gain?

For twins, you should gain 35-50 pounds during your pregnancy. It's best if you gain approximately half of that by 24 weeks.

---

costs, so it can be difficult at first to shift gears and watch those pounds pile up. Two things helped me enormously: learning about my babies' development and knowing how much they needed every calorie I could give them, and, having been so sick, realizing that all my favorite foods were finally available to me again.

People are surprised when I tell them that I love to eat, and it's a love that seems to run in my family. My mother Mieke saw to it that my sisters Sally and Anne and I all grew up with an abundance of food—really delicious, well-prepared food. Nothing thrills my sisters and me more than a fabulous restaurant, a great recipe. When we go to England for the holidays all our family celebrations are centered on food, so we bring clothing with elastic waistbands, and grow into them. Of course we all work hard to lose those holiday pounds when we get home again, but we truly do enjoy fine food.

So toward the end of the first trimester, I was happy to once again find great pleasure in food. It was so enjoyable in fact, that it didn't take me long after all to change my outlook and accept that for once, gaining weight could be a delightful goal.

How Much Should I Eat?

During your twin pregnancy, you should eat 2,700 to 3,500 calories a day, with about 20 percent of calories from protein (176 grams a day) and 40 percent each from carbohydrates and fats.

Of course when I say I enjoyed food, I don't mean I was eating French fries and ice cream all the time—although an occasional splurge on them is just fine during a twin pregnancy. This is the one time in your life when you have the green light to eat high-fat foods. You need the extra calories, so indulge! Still, if I'd eaten lower-nutrient foods all the time, pregnant or not, I know I wouldn't have had the energy to get through one of those 12-hour days on the set, much less have been able to keep going week after week. Maybe it's from years of being in show business and having to keep my energy up and my weight down, or maybe it's from my early training as a dancer, but I seem to have trained myself to love healthy foods. Salty and savory tastes, rather than rich or sweet things, attract me most. As soon as I could really eat again, I craved fish, pickles and seaweed! I stayed away from sushi though, at my doctor's request, because of the possibility of uncooked fish harboring diseases that could damage my liver. I did eat lots of other types of Asian food, which has become my favorite cuisine.

Why Am I So Tired?

Hormonal changes are the cause, along with the fact that a pregnant body simply works extremely hard all the time, even when you are resting. There's not much you can do to alleviate your fatigue besides rest! Go to bed a little earlier than usual, rest during a break at work, and try to take naps during the day if at all possible. Some women feel less tired during the second trimester, but most still need extra rest throughout their pregnancy.

Next to nausea, the crushing fatigue I felt during the first trimester was my biggest difficulty. The same is true for most women at this point, no matter what your schedule is like. We were working 12-hour days on the set of *Dr. Quinn,* and for a while I really felt I was dragging through every hour, and working hard not to show it. Beth had told me she would write my pregnancy into the story line because she'd ultimately wanted the character I played, Michaela Quinn, to have a baby anyway. But the timing wasn't quite right in the show, so I had to hide my pregnancy for the first five or six months until the show's story caught up. During that time, and as my pregnancy went on, the writers accommodated me a bit by writing episodes that were a little lighter for me so I didn't have to work quite as hard as I had been. I still needed to be in every episode, but I just wouldn't always be in every scene.

In a typical *Dr. Quinn* episode, there would be three related stories involving various characters. Normally, Dr. Quinn would be involved in two of them and she would directly influence the third. When the writers started lightening my load, Dr. Quinn would only have something to say about the third, so I didn't have to be in every shot.

Still, I was exhausted during those first months. Between scenes I'd lie down to learn my lines for the next day. Some days I'd take a nap. Other times I'd do what I eventually realized was a type of meditation—I'd sit in a chair, wide awake, and shut off all my thoughts and the sight and sounds of everything around me for a few minutes. It was very restful, and I felt I was calming myself, conserving my energy and directing it toward the babies growing inside me.

What Other Pregnancy Symptoms Should I Expect?

There are lots of blessings about having twins, and unfortunately just as many ways to feel uncomfortable during the pregnancy, too! You may not experience any of these, or you may have some or all of them to some degree (But I hope you don't!)

- **Frequent urination** as the uterus crowds your bladder.
- **Urinary tract infections** as pregnancy hormones relax the urethra and allow bacteria to travel up to the bladder.
- **An unusually keen sense of smell** which doesn't help the nausea and is the reason you can't stand your favorite perfume just now.
- **Heartburn or indigestion** as pregnancy hormones relax muscles between the stomach and esophagus.
- **Constipation** as crowding slows the action of intestines.
- **Increased heart rate and decreased blood pressure** as your blood volume increases by 40-50 percent during your pregnancy!
- **Stuffy nose and/or nosebleeds** as blood volume swells mucous membranes everywhere.
- **Overheating** as blood volume and your babies' metabolisms heat up.
- **Breast tenderness** as blood volume and pregnancy hormones increase.

Your Checkups

Eventually almost all of my own experiences with pregnancy were written into the *Dr. Quinn* series. On the show, Michaela married relatively late and worried about her age when she had difficulty getting pregnant. She even miscarried once. All of that was familiar ground to me. But Michaela and I parted company when it came to our medical care. Michaela had difficulty trusting another doctor to care for her during her pregnancy and birth. Happily, I had quite the opposite experience.

Fortunately my obstetrician, Dr. Sheryl Ross, was already experienced at caring for women pregnant with twins, so I knew I could trust her. For years she'd had two or three sets of twins in her practice at any given time. Since she was already my gynecologist, she knew James and I when we were trying desperately to get pregnant, and although we worked with Dr. Richard Paulson, a fertility specialist, she guided us and joined us on the whole roller coaster ride.

In fact, she'd been through so much with us that by the time I was pregnant, she felt almost like a member of our family. I remember that years ago, the first time I met her, she impressed me as a very intelligent woman. She just looks—and talks—like a professional, which inspired my confidence in her right away. She's taller than I am with very thick, slightly blonde hair, and she often wears a lovely pearl necklace—even when she's doing surgery! She also has what I can only describe as very beautiful laughing blue eyes. She knows when to laugh at herself—or at me! I felt completely at ease with her from the beginning, and great empathy, which I think is so important.

In fact, I would encourage you to spend some time thinking about what kind of doctor you want for this pregnancy, and then spend some time finding just the right doctor for you. Here are the things Dr. Ross and I think are most important in choosing a doctor:

1. Find a doctor who is trained and experienced in the management of high-risk pregnancies, and specifically in managing twin pregnancies.

2. Because of all the difficulties that can be part of a twin pregnancy, find a doctor who uses a team approach, with various specialists who can consult with your doctor and you on a variety of issues. For example, Dr. Ross can bring in a nutritionist, an exercise specialist, a perinatalogist (a consultant trained in high-risk obstetrics), or other specialists as they are needed when she's working with a twin pregnancy.

3. Be sure the doctor you choose has privileges at a hospital that has the facilities to take care of premature newborns, in case you need them.

4. When you have found someone who has the experience and the approach you are looking for be sure you feel comfortable talking with and asking questions of her or him.

One of the first things we did at an early checkup was set an estimated due date. Dr. Ross figured my due date by counting 40 weeks from the first day of my last period just as she would for a single pregnancy, then subtracting three weeks. She explained that about half of twins arrive around the 36th to the 38th week, which put my due date in mid- to late December. But she also stressed that I should see that date as a goal to strive toward, not something that would happen automatically. About one-third of twins are born earlier than 35 weeks, which of course can cause many complications. On that first visit, I pledged to myself that I would do my best to keep those babies safe inside me as long as I could.

That first exam was similar to initial exams when I'd had my other children. Dr. Ross wanted to know details about my medical history, my lifestyle, and my pregnancy history. Then she said she wanted to see me every two to three weeks during the first and second trimesters, and once a week during the third trimester, which is quite a bit more often than a woman pregnant with one baby is seen. But that was fine with me—I was looking forward to plenty of supervision for these babies and this pregnancy!

What to Expect at Your Checkups

- **A pelvic exam,** which should be done at your first prenatal visit, allows the doctor to examine the vagina and cervix to confirm how many weeks you are pregnant and to check for any structural problems. She should also do a Pap smear to look for any abnormal cervical changes. Usually this is done only at the first exam. At the first visit your doctor should also do a vaginal culture and chlamydia culture to check for sexually transmitted diseases or bacterial or yeast infections.

- **A urine sample** (taken at each visit) can provide signs of how well you're eating, whether you are at risk for preeclampsia (a serious complication related to blood pressure) or if you have a bladder infection.

- **A blood test** (usually done monthly) shows if you have anemia (low iron in the blood). Your blood is also evaluated early in your pregnancy for the Rh factor, which can cause problems for your babies if you are Rh negative and your partner is Rh positive. Your doctor will give you a shot of a drug called RhoGam between 26 and 28 weeks and immediately after delivery, to prevent your body from making antibodies against your babies. You should also have a RhoGam injection after any vaginal bleeding, as well as after amniocentesis. Your blood is also tested for antibodies to rubella or German measles, HIV, hepatitis B, and syphilis because these infections could be passed to your babies.

- **Weight check** to see how much weight you are gaining.

All twin pregnancies have the potential to be high risk, Dr. Ross told me, which frightened me at first. But, she explained, that doesn't mean all twin pregnancies will have things go wrong; it means that it's best to be aware of what can go wrong so it can be treated quickly. That made sense to me, and it also reassured me. My biggest risks, she said, given my age and the fact that I was carrying twins, were that I could develop hypertension of pregnancy and that I could deliver the babies too early. So her strategy from the beginning was to carefully monitor my weight gain and my blood pressure.

You may have heard similar cautions from your doctor, and I hope you will find comfort in knowing that monitoring these vital signs can go a long way toward preventing any problems. If you are in a particularly high risk category because of your age or some other issue, you may be asked to keep track of things like your blood pressure or your weight yourself at home, and you may have more frequent checkups with your doctor. In my case, there was a nurse working on the set anyway, which is standard, and Dr. Ross asked her to take my blood pressure at least once a day, and just be available if I had any questions or felt ill (other than the usual nausea that is!). That wasn't standard practice, but it was an easy thing for the nurse to do, although I confess I did feel a little embarrassed by all the fuss. In any case, the nurse faxed or telephoned Dr. Ross daily, so they were in touch all the time. Sure enough, right at the end of the first trimester my blood pressure started to elevate just a little; then the nurse practically followed me everywhere I went. Just by being constantly at my side, the nurse was my reminder to sit down and put my feet up.

By that time I had a little cooler with me all the time, and that too became a helpful reminder. It was about the size of a tool chest, and it held all the things I could eat, even when I was so nauseous. So when I had my blood pressure taken, I'd sit down, grab a snack, and put my feet up on my little cooler. Whether you're at home all day, or at the office, a personal-sized cooler like mine could do the same for you.

In my 16th week, I had amniocentesis, a prenatal test that collects genetic information about the babies. Some people elect not to have this test, although many doctors recommend it, particularly for mothers over 35. There was no question that I wanted to have the test because I wanted to know if there was a problem with the babies. But I'd had the test before, with my last pregnancy, so I knew what to expect and I knew I hated it. I have to tell you, there is nothing more frightening to me than that test. The whole idea of sticking needles into the amniotic sac is awful, but at the same time, I felt I had no choice. I had to know as much as I could about my babies.

The thing that I hadn't really thought about ahead of time was that with twins, I really had to have *two* amnios! It's one thing when they surprise you with that huge needle once, and then it's over. Somehow, psychologically I was prepared for one needle stick, because I knew it would happen suddenly and be over just as quickly. But it's quite another thing when you have to do it again, immediately. That was what I was not ready for. James was with me, which was a good thing, and I remember being more frightened during that test than I was before the birth, (when I wasn't really frightened at all!) My belly seemed so huge, but still I was scared they wouldn't find the right place for the needle without hurting the baby.

To be perfectly honest, the puncture hurts, and it is a long needle. My recommendation to anyone who's going to have amnio is, don't look at the needle! You really don't want to know about that needle. Think of something to visualize, have someone with you to look at, bring a lovely picture—a photo of two babies, or of your other children. But don't look at the needle!

Once the needle is in, I'm happy to say it's no longer painful and it is actually fun to follow what the doctor is doing on the ultrasound screen. I watched the whole thing both times, which was reassuring and actually quite fascinating.

Prenatal Tests You May Choose in the First Trimester (Weeks 1–12)

Amniocentesis is a way of collecting samplings of genetic material from the amniotic fluid, where as fetuses grow, they discard cells. If you choose to have this test, it is performed between 15 and 20 weeks gestation, and involves a long needle. Guided by ultrasound, the needle is inserted into the uterus where a small amount of amniotic fluid from each baby's sac is withdrawn. The fluid is analyzed for chromosomal abnormalities and the babies' gender is determined. You can choose whether or not you want to be told your babies' genders.

Chorionic villus sampling (CVS) is a way of collecting samplings of genetic material from the babies earlier than amniocentesis. Between the 10th and 12th week of pregnancy, a long thin needle guided by ultrasound is inserted either through the uterus or through the vagina and cervix to the chorion, a membrane that eventually becomes part of the placenta. Villi, tiny projections on the chorion contain the baby's genetic material. The samplings are analyzed and results are available within about two weeks.

Your Babies, As They Grow

I absolutely loved seeing my babies on ultrasound, even at the very beginning when they looked like no more than two tiny dark blips in a field of snowy static. If you're sure it's twins, you've probably already had at least one ultrasound, so you'll know what I mean when I say that seeing those babies, even on that fuzzy ultrasound screen, makes the pregnancy very real, very immediate. In addition to seeing Dr. Ross, we went to a perinatologist, Dr. Connie Agnew, early on, who used a high resolution ultrasound which showed more detail than the typical ultrasound. It was the most amazing machine. It seemed she could literally count every finger, every hair, and every eyelash on each baby. It was amazing what she could find. She'd look at every organ, the heart, the kidneys, look at the size and measure each for their growth, even when the boys were tiny. James and I were enormously reassured seeing those ultrasounds, because we could be certain the boys were growing well, that everything was forming correctly. We saw Dr. Agnew three or four times and then continued with the standard ultrasounds at Dr. Ross' office, which I then had every three weeks. By the way, when you're pregnant with twins, it's typical to have ultrasounds more frequently than your girlfriends who may have one or two ultrasounds during their whole pregnancy.

Because of all those highly detailed ultrasounds, it seems like we've always known that we had two boys. I didn't mind knowing their genders ahead of time, and to be honest, I was much more concerned about miscarrying than I was about being surprised by their genders when they were born. For some couples keeping the gender secret from friends and family, or not being told themselves, is an important issue. For us it was not. I suppose gender was just another piece of information about them, like knowing they had five fingers on each hand and that their kidneys were developing well. I think also because we'd each had children before, which gender we had didn't really matter to us either. Healthy babies were our only concern.

No matter which machine we used, it was always a welcome sight to peek in at those two little guys safe inside my tummy. Seeing how much they'd change from one ultrasound appointment to the next was all I needed to keep my spirits up when I thought I

Is Ultrasound Safe for My Babies?

It's safe to say that the answer is yes. Many studies have been conducted since ultrasound was first used in the 1950s to find the definitive answer to this question. In 1988, the American Institute of Ultrasound in Medicine Bioeffects Committee concluded that the use of ultrasound produced "no confirmed biological effects on patients . . ." Today, nearly 80 percent of American women have at least one ultrasound during pregnancy.

---

couldn't face another queasy morning or one more saltine. James and I would come away from each appointment dazzled, awestruck once again by what a miracle these babies were.

Very early on we began referring to the blips as This One and That One. "Look!" I'd say to James, "this one seems so patient and calm and that one is always moving." As James often says now, that was a creative time for us in more ways than the obvious. Our conversations and observations about This One and That One were what sparked the idea for our series of children's books by the same name. After the boys were born, we were fascinated to see that the personalities that we'd observed in them long before they were born were—and still are—the personalities we see in them now. Kris ("That One") is the one who, even in the early ultrasounds was always moving about, bouncing and wriggling. Today, he's the taller, more physical one, more of a daredevil. And Johnny, he's the careful one, the one more likely to sit down with an art project or a book, the one more likely to play quietly on his own for a while.

How Your Babies Grow During the First Trimester

For the first three months, the growth of twins is similar to that of a single baby in the womb:

- **Weeks 4–8:** The spinal cord and nervous system, the heart and circulatory system of each baby, still called an embryo, is developing. By the end of this period, each will also have the beginnings of all major organs, as well as arms, hands, finger buds, and legs and feet. Eyes are clearly defined.

- **Weeks 8–12:** This is the start of a major growth period that will last through week 20. By week 10, the embryos will have taken on a much more human look and they are officially called fetuses. Organs and limbs continue to be defined.

- **Weeks 12–16:** The babies are moving around more, practicing breathing movements, extending their fingers, and waving their arms and legs. Toward the end of the period you may be able to feel their movements. You also may be able to tell your babies' genders on an ultrasound scan.

Your Self, Your Family

During my pregnancy I painted watercolors a great deal, and it was a tremendous joy to me. You might think that it sounds crazy to fit one more activity into a schedule already so crowded. But I know you'll understand when I say that it was the one thing I really did for myself alone. Painting has a calming influence on me, like playing the piano does for some people, or meditating or praying or writing in a journal does for others. When I'm painting, my hands are busy but my mind floats free, so it's rejuvenating, refreshing, even restful in its own way.

If you have an activity that makes you feel that way, I hope you'll try to make time for it during your pregnancy. If you don't have an activity like that, I would highly recommend that you find one! It's so easy to become overwhelmed with the importance and perhaps the difficulties of a twin pregnancy. The little bits of time you spend pampering yourself will only add to your sense of well-being. And, there are those who believe calming yourself adds to your babies' well-being too.

I had painted as a child, and studied art in high school, and then I hadn't done art of any kind until I was 40. When I did, it was because my life was falling apart. I was going through a miserable divorce, and my accountant had told me I'd probably have to declare bankruptcy. An antidote to all the unhappiness was to spend time with my children, Katie and Sean, who were very young. We'd finger-paint together in the playroom for hours. At this time I attended a charity event I'd been invited to, and the only thing I could afford to purchase as a donation to the charity was the services of an artist to do a drawing of my children. When he came to the house to take photos of them for the drawing, he noticed the fingerpaintings. I told him they were mine, and he suggested I take up painting! Although I liked playing with paint, I really didn't know much about formal painting techniques, and he volunteered to teach me how to do watercolor.

The next thing I knew it became the driving force of my life. I just couldn't stop painting. I drew and painted all day and all night—obsessively. And I rediscovered the joy I got from art. The amazing thing was that with all the pain and frustration I was going through, what came out in my art was the most tranquil paintings. It seemed the more upset I was, the more tranquil the paintings were. It was fascinating.

Like you, I seldom have long stretches of unscheduled time in which I can just sit down and do something I love. So I was always lugging my art box with me to the set, painting a little here and a little there when I found I had a few moments between scenes. Finally someone from the props department set up a lovely little painting table for me, which I used almost every day. Of course in the middle of a busy set it seemed there was always someone peering over my shoulder, watching me paint.

While taking care of yourself has to be a priority on many levels during your pregnancy, if you have other children, they have to be high on your list too. It's important to prepare them for the arrival of the babies; especially when there will be two or more babies to contend with. James and I talked with Katie and Sean about adding to our family well before I was pregnant, and they were completely excited and all for it.

Once I was pregnant though, I quickly saw how easily they might feel eclipsed. Nothing about the pregnancy was ordinary, and it was clear that life itself would never again be ordinary after the babies were born. Already, early in my pregnancy, there were an enormous number of gifts being sent to the house for the babies. The whole world seemed excited I was having twins, long before they were born. I could already see that twins of any age—infants, toddlers, or older—would always command more attention than a single child would.

So I set about to find a way to be sure Katie and Sean still felt special. The first thing I did was to go upstairs to my memorabilia room, a large closet, really, just off the gym, which is crammed full of photos and other special items. I spent hours in there, pulling out all my favorite baby pictures of Katie and Sean, and of Kalen, James' grown son, and Jenni, my ex-husband's daughter who spent lots of time with us. There were a few I didn't want to permanently remove from their albums, so I had color copies made of those. Most were just family favorites, but there were some magazine covers for various women's magazines I'd done with Katie or with Sean. Then I gathered all the pictures up and headed for the kitchen, where I assembled a rather large display of everyone's baby pictures on the refrigerator and the counter next to it. Everyone loved seeing themselves as babies again, and I think it really

The Straight Scoop:
Notes for Dads from James

Pregnancy, especially at the beginning, can seem like it's only about the woman, and some men feel kind of left out. During Jane's pregnancy, I learned that while physically, it *is* all happening to the woman, pregnancy is really about the couple. You're half of the equation, and what she needs now is for you to hold up your half.

It's an amazing thing to watch the extraordinary hormonal changes a pregnant woman goes through. If you're not part of the process, participating, taking care of her, a man can become part of the problem.

The most important thing a man can do for his wife at this time is to tell her how excited he is that these babies are coming. I know you may be nervous about it, worried about how you'll handle all this financially, emotionally. And it's good to have honest conversations about these things. But know when to stop. It's really hard on a woman who's literally carrying the weight of the pregnancy to keep hearing about your apprehension and fears. These babies are a great gift to you. Your gift in return is to really learn to love someone more than yourself, and then act accordingly.

helped each of the kids recall that they too, had been the center of attention, and even famous, when they were babies. You could do the same thing, displaying baby photos of your own grown children anywhere they will be seen constantly—in the kitchen, an entryway or a corridor.

Jane's pregnancy was a time of tremendous emotional highs and occasionally, some pretty deep lows. Luckily, she was able to funnel a lot of the emotional energy that comes with early pregnancy into her work as an actress. If your wife doesn't have that kind of built-in emotional outlet, you could be seeing those extreme ups-and-downs, and you're probably not used to them. Here's what I did when that happened with Jane: I'd just take a deep breath and remember what my conscience had told me—"Whatever she says is right."

Generally speaking, during stressful times early in the pregnancy, I tried to make sure that anything Jane needed, in any way, shape or form, was taken care of. Any stress I could foresee, I kept away from her as best I could. I knew that if Dr. Ross told Jane she had to stop working immediately for the babies' sake, she would make that sacrifice because the babies meant everything. But in the meantime, life went on, and I saw it as my job to keep day-to-day stress away from Jane.

I see my role—the man's role—as being of service to those he loves, as creating harmony as much as possible, and learning patience. Pregnancy is a great time to practice what it is to be a father, learning that patience and practicing that creation of harmony.

After the boys were born, I continued to update the collection to correspond with their age, and it's been a fun retrospective of our family. Now, for example, the boys are in preschool, and I have displayed several photos of Katie and Sean at that age, (Jenni and Kalen are grown and gone). One favorite that has stayed out in the kitchen is a shot of me playing Marie Antoinette, with Katie as the queen's daughter and Sean as the young Dauphin—he was only four at the time—all elegantly dressed in pale blue.

We've all enjoyed those pictures so much, I've been thinking of making color copies of all of them and creating small albums for each child, filled with a few favorite photos from each year from birth to their current age.

Looking Good, Feeling Good

Looking good while I was pregnant with twins had more to do with sanity than with vanity. Because I'd had two miscarriages right before this pregnancy, to say I was worried at first would be putting it lightly. I was terrified and I badly needed to find some balance in my life so I didn't fret constantly about the possibility of losing these babies. If I'd had nothing else to do but worry, I would have certainly lost my mind. Usually, I'm much better off if I can focus on doing something rather than focusing on *not* doing something. So I made it my job to do two things: first and foremost, I would do everything I could to support this pregnancy. That was my number one priority beyond everything else.

Second: I decided I would focus on being extremely healthy by eating well and exercising appropriately. The payoff would be not only that I was actively doing things to help the pregnancy, but also that I would look as good as I could, for as long as I could. After all, before getting pregnant, I had promised everyone I worked with that I didn't usually look pregnant until I was quite far along, even showing off photos from my previous pregnancies to prove my point. But I hadn't counted on twins!

Once I saw looking good as a challenging part of an important job—producing healthy babies—then it became fun and interesting to keep up with, and adapt to all the physical changes that go along with being pregnant with twins. As my body, my hair and my skin changed, I simply set out to find new approaches to each new set of challenges. Maybe most important, I was constantly reminded that all these changes were temporary. I turned to just about anyone I could think of for help, professional consultants and friends alike. Looking back, I can honestly say that throughout my pregnancy, I did feel much more attractive and had much less trouble adapting to my growing body than I'd thought I would. Everyone's pregnancy is different, but I hope some of the things that worked for me, will work for you, too.

Exercise

I imagined, correctly so, that with twins, I'd pop out in front much quicker than I had with either of my single babies. Still, I vowed at least to maintain the muscle tone in my arms and legs and the muscles that support my posture. I wanted to learn how best to walk, sit, and stand to help my body to support the weight that would come with two babies. I'd also had terrible back pain with my other pregnancies, so I knew that had to be taken into account in planning any kind of exercise program.

The idea of exercising through a pregnancy was familiar to me. I had exercised during both of my other pregnancies. In fact, I'd been on the cover of a pregnancy exercise book—*Jane Fonda's Pregnancy Workout*. I hadn't intended to. In fact, I had driven miles out of my way, from my Beverly Hills home to a studio in the San Fernando Valley to attend classes at a studio where I was not likely to be known. I didn't want to be notorious, so it was funny when Femmy deLeyser, the woman who wrote the book and conducted our classes asked me if I'd be one of the people photographed both inside the book and on the cover. She didn't choose me because I was an actress; in fact she didn't know who I was until after she chose me for the cover. She told me she chose me because I was balletic and looked good doing the exercises. When we shot the cover, I was the only one of the group who hadn't given birth yet. They needed someone who was still pregnant, someone who'd just delivered, Femmy, and Jane Fonda. When we all showed up for the shoot, Jane turned to me and said, "Don't I know you?" It was a funny moment.

Looking balletic even when I was pregnant seemed to come naturally to me. In a sense, I had trained to be a dancer from the time I was a very small child (my mother says I danced before I walked!). Ballet was my passion; as a child I wanted to be a ballerina more than life itself. I had no interest in anything else—just classical music or music I could turn into a ballet. At the age of 13 I enrolled in a professional ballet school, the School of the Arts Educational Trust in London. But by the time I was 17, I'd injured my knees so badly I was told I'd never be a ballerina. I was crushed, but I immediately segued into the acting program at the school, which I also loved.

I regret now that I gave up dancing so quickly and completely. There were other types of dancing I probably could have done that wouldn't have involved the same stresses as ballet. But I do know that whatever figure I have now must be credited to that training.

That's why, even pregnant with twins, I assumed I would work out in some way. But of course I was concerned about safety—that of the babies as well as mine. When I asked her, Dr. Ross immediately assured me that a correctly *modified* exercise program was absolutely necessary, even for a fit mother of twins. She put me in touch with Birgitta Gallo, a personal trainer who had worked with pregnant women, and with whom she had written a book called *Expecting Fitness,* to develop that program. I'd always exercised on my own, never with a personal trainer, so that idea was new to me. But I knew that between the two of them, they were the experts, and I was prepared to listen to, and heed, everything they had to say.

I was fortunate to have these two experts guiding me every step of the way. If you don't already have an arrangement like this in place, I would say that **before you decide whether you should initiate an exercise program or continue what you've been doing, you must check with your doctor!** Then, because you won't have Birgitta by your side, I would encourage you to either join a class at your local recreation center, health club or YMCA that is offered specifically for pregnant women or better yet, for women who are pregnant with twins. If you like to work with a trainer, the YMCA often offers that service at a reasonable cost. In any case, please clear any exercise program with your doctor before you proceed.

Because of my history of miscarriages, I didn't exercise at all during my first trimester, other than Kegels and a fair amount of walking I naturally did on the set. Birgitta and I began our work in the second trimester.

Should You Exercise?

If you have had miscarriages, your doctor may recommend you wait until the second trimester to see if exercising will be appropriate for you then. Even if you have been exercising right along, with twins, you will need to modify what you are doing. Check with your doctor about modifications.

However, if your doctor gives the go-ahead, your body will function best when you exercise regularly.

Here is a basic exercise program for pregnancy:

Warm-up: 5–10 minutes (walking, stair machine, stationary bike).

Low-stress aerobics: 25–45 minutes 3 to 6 days a week. Choose a special prenatal aerobics class, or an activity you enjoy, such as swimming, walking briskly, or using a low-impact machine like a stair machine, elliptical trainer, or stationary bike.

Toning: 20–60 minutes, 2 to 3 days a week. Focus on strengthening the pelvic floor (with Kegels), and the abdominals.

Cool down: 5–10 minutes of gentle stretching.

Exercise Guidelines for Pregnant Women

The American College of Obstetricians and Gyne-
cologists issued these guidelines in 1994 for pregnant women. While they are intended for women
carrying a single baby, they provide a good starting
point for understanding how to safely exercise
during your pregnancy. (Parentheses and italics are
author's addition for emphasis.)

- There is no need to limit exercise intensity and
  lower target heart rate unless the woman *has
  risk factors that could compromise her pregnancy (such as a twin pregnancy or previous
  miscarriages.)* She should have a health assess-
  ment and an individualized exercise program.
- Regular exercise (at least three times a week) at
  mild to moderate intensities is better than spo-
  radic exercise.
- The supine (lying on your back) position after
  the first trimester is not advisable. Neither is
  standing still for a long time.

Most doctors consider a twin pregnancy a high-risk pregnancy by definition. In discussing what I would be doing once I
did begin to exercise, Dr. Ross stressed that my exercise program
would carefully focus on maintaining muscle tone and helping
support the weight of the pregnancy, including building strength
in my back. I'd be working on upper and lower back muscles,
abdominal muscles, and the muscles of the pelvic floor.

The one exercise she said it was fine to do even in the first
trimester was Kegels. If you've had children already, you know
about Kegels. You may also know that they are *so* important in

- Exercise should be halted if the woman is fatigued, because she has less available oxygen with which to do aerobic exercise. It is also not recommended to exercise to exhaustion.
- Weight-bearing exercises, such as walking and running, may be continued throughout pregnancy, but with caution. Non-weight-bearing exercises, such as cycling and swimming, minimize the risk of injury and so can be continued throughout the pregnancy.
- Exercises that compromise a woman's balance, or have the potential of causing abdominal trauma, should be avoided. This is especially true for the third trimester.
- Eating more than the 300–500 extra calories a day (*or more, per baby*) that the pregnancy needs is advisable if the woman exercises regularly.
- Drinking a lot of water, wearing clothes that breathe, and avoiding hot and humid weather when exercising is advisable.

helping to avoid one particularly miserable postpartum surprise—lack of bladder control. Named for Dr. Arnold Kegel, the exercise strengthens the pelvic floor muscles and you can do it anywhere, any time without anyone knowing! Birgitta taught me to first visualize the pelvic floor, then to alternately squeeze and relax the muscles around the anus, then the vagina. Then, squeeze and pull the muscles of the perineum (the space between the anus and vagina) in and up, exhaling as you squeeze, inhaling as you release. Do five at a time, holding each one for five to 10 seconds.

Dressing Well

I was lucky to have a lot of help in this area. Cheri Ingle, the costume designer for *Dr. Quinn* was indispensable. In addition to designing Dr. Quinn clothing that would hide my pregnancy at first, she ended up picking out or actually making a lot of my real life clothing. Overall, what she did for me worked so well, I wanted to pass it on. In fact I wish I could wave a magic wand and produce a personal stylist for every woman pregnant with twins. That may seem frivolous, but I think you'll agree that this is when we all need the most help in dressing ourselves!

Because Cheri's primary mission was to keep me looking the least pregnant for the longest time possible for the show, she started with subtle adaptations to our usual costumes so that overall, I would have the same silhouette. You might keep similar goals in mind for your own wardrobe. First, she made a new line of skirts a little bigger than my normal size—not even a whole size larger. If you aren't fitting into your clothing, this could be a guide for you. You may not need maternity clothing, but a few new pieces one size larger might do for a while, or you might add a couple of basic pieces to your wardrobe in one of the new stretchy fabrics. They're very comfortable and while no one likes to buy clothes they won't wear for long, it beats buying a maternity wardrobe before you need it. I also like empire-waist dresses; they emphasize the bust not the waist! I've found too that some of the non-maternity clothing I wore early in my pregnancy was perfect for me to wear in the first weeks after the boys were born. I didn't want to wear maternity clothing, but I didn't quite fit into my own clothing, so those pieces allowed me to make some useful compromises.

You might be able to make your current wardrobe work for a little longer with a couple of tricks Cheri used on my costumes. She added a bit of elastic at the waist on the side, just a simple casing with a little elastic in it. And she sewed three buttons on the waistband of each skirt, reasoning that when you're pregnant, most women can bloat up some days, and not on others. One day I might button it on the first button, the next day on the third. The elastic and button adjustments were easy—I did them on some pieces in my personal wardrobe—and they contributed enormously to my being as comfortable as possible. It was summer then, and we were working through long, hot days. Seeing me sweat through 14 hours of shooting wearing petticoats, tights, a voluminous skirt, a shirt, maybe a jacket, Cheri told me she felt really dedicated to making me as comfortable as she could. And I truly appreciated her efforts!

Is It Time to Buy Maternity Clothes?

You can expect that, since it's carrying two babies, your uterus will be bigger than that of your girl-friend who is carrying one baby. It probably won't be twice as big, but it could be about half again the size of hers. Does this mean you'll need maternity clothes at 16 weeks? That's hard to say. It depends on things like how your body is carrying the babies, the size of your pre-pregnant body, and how accommodating your non-maternity wardrobe is!

In my personal wardrobe, I did what a lot of women do. I wore some of James' shirts or an over-sized sweater over tights. Although I did poke out sooner than in my other pregnancies, thankfully I didn't have to make huge changes in my personal wardrobe until the second trimester. The fact that I spent my days on the set and seldom needed to go out in my own clothing, had a lot to do with that!

Details

One of the biggest bonuses for being pregnant is this: no matter what your hair was like before, for the next nine months it will grow faster and feel thicker than ever. I don't know all the scientific explanations for it, but I imagine it has to do with the pregnancy hormones, your nutrition, and the fact that your body is just growing everything!

If you have not had long hair before, this might be a great time to try growing yours out. I've always chosen to have long hair because I feel I have more variation when it's long. I can tie it back or I can have it loose and long, or I can have lots of other combinations of up and down, straight or curled.

Can I Dye My Hair or Get a Perm When I'm Pregnant?

The chemical solutions used in permanents and dyes are absorbed through the scalp and into the bloodstream. Still, studies have shown that neither has detrimental effects on the fetus. Breathing the fumes from some solutions might be a problem though, and in general it's a good idea to avoid them until the second trimester.

Some women say that perms don't always take evenly when you are pregnant, and you could end up with an unpleasant combination of straight and curly locks. Another reason to consider waiting until after the pregnancy to curl.

If you're considering cutting your hair very short anyway during your pregnancy because you hope it will be easier to care for, I'd urge you to think first about proportion. Short hair may be right for you, but I did feel that my long hair sort of balanced out the size of my body as I got bigger. There may be someone who looks good with really short hair and a very large belly, but I knew it wasn't going to be me!

Many women, and I'm one of them, also felt that their skin took on a lovely glow during their pregnancy. My doctor told me it was the increased blood volume that added that rosy sheen, but whatever it was, I enjoyed it thoroughly. Not everyone gets that glow however. I hope you're one who does, but please be forewarned that some women just look a little washed-out and tired during their pregnancy. Others find that their skin takes on some adolescent characteristics and breaks out. You may find that you have to revamp your skin care routine to accommodate these changes.

I hate to be the bearer of yet another piece of unpleasant news, but there is one more skin change everyone worries about: stretch marks. I'm amazed that after three pregnancies, the few I had have all disappeared. During my first pregnancy I bought all the products like vitamin E and various creams that were supposed to prevent stretch marks and was religious about using them. My second pregnancy I occasionally remembered to use them. By the third pregnancy, I realized I'd just been lucky. I've heard it said that the surest way to avoid stretch marks is to choose your parents well, but my mother and sisters all have them. So I'm afraid I have no great wisdom to pass on about how to avoid stretch marks. But I do know that even though they can look red and very obvious at first, they do fade with time and can eventually be barely noticeable. I like the attitude of one friend whose belly still bears the subtle silvery lines left by her pregnancy. She calls those stretch marks her "badge of honor" for having given birth to twins!

Stretch marks or no, I also found it felt good to keep my belly moisturized as it grew, and smoothing on a good cream with vitamin E in it felt lovely after a shower or bath.

As you come to the end of early pregnancy, I hope all the discomforts and adjustments are also coming to a close for you. Lots of people feel that mid-pregnancy is the best time of all. You should have your energy back, and you'll probably be feeling more confident and secure in the pregnancy. If you're not there yet, you can know that you do have many wonderful days to look forward to!

Checklist for Early Pregnancy

Begin:

- Eating as well as you can.
- Gaining about 1–1½ pounds a week.
- Taking a daily prenatal multivitamin supplement that has 30–60 mg of iron and .4 mg of folic acid. You should also be getting 1200 mg a day of calcium. In addition, 200 ug/d of chromium can help prevent gestational diabetes later in the pregnancy.
- Checking with your doctor about exercising at all or modifying your exercise plan.
- Napping when you're tired.
- Drinking 8 glasses of water each day.
- Thinking about childbirth preparation classes. Because your pregnancy will likely be 36–38 weeks rather than 40 weeks, consider starting classes and selecting a hospital within the next few weeks.
- Relaxing into your pregnancy!

Stop:

- Using caffeine.
- Drinking alcohol.
- Smoking; avoid second hand smoke.
- Dieting to lose weight.
- Taking over-the-counter drugs for colds or allergies without consulting your doctor first.

three

Living in a Different World

Weeks 17–28

Ah, the middle months of pregnancy. This is where life becomes smoother as your belly becomes larger! I remember thinking that the first three months of my twin pregnancy had been like a sometimes-scary ride on a bumpy, unfamiliar back road, carrying me to a foreign world where I didn't speak the language or know the customs. Everything was a bit of a surprise, and it simply took a little while to adjust to each one.

But by the fourth month or so, I started to get comfortable in the world I occupied. I don't mean to say that I was often actually *comfortable* in a body that continued to grow and change by the minute! What I mean is that I knew more about what to expect from myself and from the pregnancy, and there was comfort in that.

As you enter this relatively calm mid-pregnancy world, I hope you too will know the comfort that comes with a certain amount of predictability.

Your Pregnant Body

Perhaps the best news of all about mid-pregnancy is that eating can become a joy again. For most women—myself included—the nausea finally goes away. I can't give you a specific day when it will vanish, because that's different for everyone. Some women find that nausea doesn't *completely* disappear, but that it does diminish. In my mind, anything less than vomiting all day is heaven. The fatigue I felt for the first three months had, for the most part, gone too, and I usually felt wonderful. At work, I felt like my old self, just a little larger in the tummy! I did slow down a bit, however, just to be on the safe side. I didn't always work the entire day, and I often worked a slightly shorter week than usual—five or six out of the seven days it took to shoot one episode.

On a typical day I'd still arrive at the set at 5:45 A.M. and go directly to the hair and makeup trailer, except now there were no plastic buckets to lug and no constant threat of being sick. I'd have breakfast during the hour and a half it took to do my hair and makeup. Now that I could really eat again, I concentrated on protein and anything that was dense in nutrients. The caterers were very good about being sure I got the food I needed, and each day they made me a special breakfast, which they called the Jane Omelet. It was an egg white omelet with lots of vegetables such as mushrooms, onions, and green peppers. And it had white cheese—no yellow, artificially colored, processed cheese. They'd put some bacon on the plate and I'd nibble the lean parts, just for flavor. Then I'd eat the crispy parts of the hash browns, never the soft inside—I only like the crispy part. Sometimes they'd add a piece of whole-wheat toast, and there was always some fresh fruit. It was a big breakfast, but I needed it—it gave me the energy I always needed for my work.

Sometimes, in the middle of my breakfast, the crew would be lighting a scene and I'd have to run to the set with my hair half in rollers, my makeup half done—and my breakfast half eaten. I'm sure I looked a sight! By that time *Dr. Quinn* had been on for a

What If Eating Still Isn't Fun?

Heartburn happens to most pregnant women at one time or another because pregnancy hormones relax the esophageal sphincter, the little muscle that usually keeps stomach contents from back flowing into the esophagus. Women pregnant with twins tend to get heartburn earlier and more frequently than women pregnant with one baby. What can you do? Stay away from spicy foods, try not to overeat, and don't lie down after a meal. You might even try propping yourself up at night at about a 45-degree angle to keep your esophagus higher than your stomach. Tums antacid tablets work well for most women, but if they don't work for you, check with your doctor about using a liquid antacid, which will coat the esophageal lining more effectively. As a bonus, they also provide some extra calcium.

If you are still feeling nauseous or vomiting after the 12th week of pregnancy let your doctor know. She can help you prevent nutritional deficiencies, weight loss and dehydration. Try drinking small amounts of very cold liquids such as ginger ale or lemon-lime soda through a straw (to minimize the amount of air you take in). Or eat small amounts of solid foods such as crackers, dry toast, cereal or baked potatoes every couple of hours. Keep a food diary for a while, recording everything you eat and how you feel afterwards, to ferret out the culprits upsetting your stomach.

couple of years, and lots of fans came to the set to watch us shoot. Those fans ended up with a pretty intimate view of me in various stages of dress and undress, my hair askew and no makeup! In any case, once the lighting was set, I always managed to zip back to the trailer to finish my Jane Omelet.

At lunch and dinner, I'd have fish or chicken with rice or potatoes and lots of vegetables. I love spicy food, so if my usual fare could be prepared with plenty of spice, I was particularly happy until heartburn set in. Although I tended to get heartburn from spicy foods during my pregnancy, sometimes I ate it anyway, just for the joy of tasting it!

Between meals I'd nibble on protein bars and a particular type of frozen fruit bar that I loved. Smoothies made with yogurt, fruit

---

Can I Eat Sushi When I'm Pregnant? How About Fast Food?

Say goodbye to sushi for a while. Generally speaking, you should avoid raw, undercooked fish and shellfish that might have been improperly refrigerated, including sushi. They increase your risk of exposure to Salmonella, parasites and hepatitis A infection, each of which can damage your liver. To lower your risk even further, make sure all meats and fish are cooked to an internal temperature of 160 degrees. If you really can't live without sushi for a while, stick to vegetable-only rolls.

Fast food isn't a total no-no, but it is generally high in sodium and in fat, so use your discretion. If you are having difficulty gaining weight, stopping off for a burger every now and then may help. But keep in mind that your overall goal should be to eat high quality calories more often than not.

and protein powder were great too. I drank a lot of cranberry juice, diluted with water. I knew I needed a lot of water anyway, and this made drinking it easier. I didn't get bladder infections, as some women do when they are pregnant, but I felt it was sort of a precaution. The cranberry juice kept me from drinking diet soda as well, which I didn't want to drink.

In all, this was a good time for me as far as drinking and eating were concerned. I was able to eat anything, and I did eat a wide variety of healthy foods, but I still felt I was working hard to gain weight.

One of the hardest parts of eating properly was fitting meal-times into my erratic workday. The production people and writers continued to try to schedule me a little lighter, but there was so much pressure to finish each episode on time, that it was hard to make huge changes in the schedule. I did have my old energy back, so it wasn't too difficult except when we had to shoot at night. Our normal schedule for daytime shooting would go from 5:45 or so in the morning until 5:00 or 6:00 in the evening. But when we were scheduled to shoot night scenes, sometimes we'd start at 6:00 or 7:00 in the evening and get home at 8:00 the next morning! Those extreme schedule changes were quite exhausting to me, and I always made sure I had the following day off. Other days we'd start at 10 A.M. and have lunch at 4 P.M. and shoot into the evening, which wasn't so difficult. It all depended on what kind of light the story demanded.

I know many women work odd shifts like this. If you find yourself in that situation, I would urge you to be particularly careful about getting what you and your babies need—enough rest and healthy food. On the set, I made certain I always took breaks on the same schedule I would have if we were shooting on a regular daytime schedule—every six hours. I could put my feet up and eat a meal. Of course I also snacked constantly and drank lots of water as I did during the day. Still, I had to be very careful to keep track of what I had eaten and when, so that I didn't inadvertently skip a meal. No matter whether the clock said it was traditional mealtime or not, I'd be sure to have my three meals and three snacks according to the schedule I was working.

Although work could be difficult during this time, I consoled myself with the knowledge that I knew my bottom line—that I would protect the health and well-being of my babies above all else—and I knew I would act accordingly. I measured everything I did against that standard.

Do You Have Anemia?

Almost everyone who's pregnant with twins becomes anemic, so even if you've never been anemic before, you should watch for the signs now. You'll be pale, extremely tired, and you'll feel weak. You might have heart palpitations, shortness of breath and even fainting spells.

Of course you can take iron supplements (between meals), but ask your doctor to help you find one that won't be constipating. You can also eat iron-rich foods such as red meats. Stay away from caffeine, milk and tea when taking iron supplements because they interfere with its absorption.

By the time I was four or five months pregnant, I definitely looked like I was at least six months along. I was grateful I spent most of my time within a sort of closed community on the set. Everyone knew me, knew when I was due, so I didn't have to answer a lot of silly, repetitive questions. When I was out somewhere else, it was another story. I soon learned how annoying it could be to be barraged with personal questions from people you don't know. I am used to being interviewed, and I know the ground rules there. But somehow I felt different about talking about my pregnancy when I was out socially. Someone I didn't know well would invariably ask, "When are you due?" or, "How far along are you?" Then I would have to spend ten minutes explaining that, yes, I was sure of my due date even though it looked like I should be due sooner, and yes, I knew it was twins, and then they'd want to know if I used fertility drugs and on and on. People can ask the most personal questions just because you're having twins! You don't have to be a celebrity to feel badgered by a curious person who wants to know more about your private life than you wish to tell.

During this time I felt it was particularly important to hold to my philosophy that while any twin pregnancy is rather public because you look so obviously pregnant, the details of one's life are private. I was even tempted to avoid altogether the issue of what was private and what wasn't by simply saying I was due sooner than I was, because of the size of my belly. I didn't do that; I don't like dishonesty, and it would have been more complicated in the end anyway. But I did get to the point that I just didn't feel I had to go into detail with people I didn't know well. I got pretty good at politely deflecting questions I didn't want to answer by saying things like, "Oh that's such a long story . . ." and then quickly changing the subject.

The size of my belly, which grew so large so quickly, was an issue for me in other ways too. A big one was balance; I kept toppling over! I never had a problem with balance in my other pregnancies. I used to be a ballerina, for goodness sake! I could stand on one toe and count to 20. Now however, I could be on *terra firma* wearing good sensible shoes and I was unnerved to find myself losing my balance all the time. Most often I would just stumble and catch myself. But once when we were shooting at the *Dr. Quinn* homestead, I was standing on the rather steep front steps doing a scene and I lurched and then literally toppled over. I remember two people came running to catch me—one was Joe Lando who played Sully—and I thought, "Thank goodness it's two of them!" No damage was done, thankfully. When he heard about my adventure later in the day, James said my lack of balance was because my body had outgrown my feet, which are a rather small size 6. There's probably some truth to that!

Why Do I Feel So Unsteady on My Feet?

Many women feel unsteady when they are pregnant with one baby, much less pregnant with twins—and for good reason. Not only is your center of gravity likely to be different because of your growing belly, but pregnancy hormones also loosen all your ligaments. So, while it is harder than usual to keep your balance, it's also easier than usual to turn your ankle. Now is the time to watch your step and wear flat shoes!

Usually, we took a break from shooting the show during the summer, which was one of the reasons I liked doing the series—I could be off work while my children were home from school. This year though, because of my pregnancy, we continued to shoot right through the summer to get as many of the following season's episodes finished as we could before I had to stop working. This schedule also assured that I would get about six weeks off after the twins were born. My due date was December 20. I'd planned to take a couple of weeks off before that, and Beth assured me that we could adjust the beginning of the shooting schedule in late January if necessary to be sure I had enough time to recuperate. It was the same type of juggling act you may be facing if you are trying to plan your pregnancy leave to fit your work schedule. Plus, I had the added concern that during this trimester it was becoming increasingly difficult to hide my pregnancy, and my character wasn't pregnant yet.

The last episode in which we had to hide it was called "The Expedition," and it was the most physically demanding one I ever did. In the episode, a group of women characters and I were proving that women could climb Pikes Peak as well as men, so we were all dressed in "men's clothing," meaning heavy wool trousers. I also wore a flannel shirt and a heavy jacket to hide my belly. Temperatures were in the 90s and above every day, and we were all sweltering. We actually hiked quite a ways the day we shot those scenes, and although at the time I felt strong enough and able to do the scene, afterwards, I was tired enough to know that I probably shouldn't have done it. During breaks I would lie down on a portable chaise lounge, drink ice water and rest. Needless to say, I got through it, but I certainly wouldn't recommend women pregnant with twins to do anything remotely similar!

Looking back, I think it was not a good decision on my part to participate as fully as I did in that scene and I feel some remorse about that. I did it because I felt this huge responsibility, as we all do toward friends and family who rely on us. There were over 200 people working on my show, and they all—crew and cast—felt like family to me. In a very real sense, I was responsible for their jobs. If I didn't do *my* job, I was so scared people would think I'd let them down, and if we lost the series because of my pregnancy, I actually would have let them down. On the other hand, looking at this situation now, I know that if I'd lost the babies because of my sense of responsibility to the show I would have never forgiven myself. So I have to admit that this was a mistake. Bolstered by the fact that I felt all right while I was doing the scene, I can see now that I took a risk that I really shouldn't have. I am just so grateful that I was lucky enough that my babies did not pay the price for it.

Here was an issue I juggled constantly—balancing my responsibility to the babies I was carrying with my responsibility to the people who worked on my show. The only way I could resolve these issues was to keep coming back to my bottom line—that I would do what was best for my babies. I'm sorry to say that wasn't always perfectly clear, and I wasn't always perfectly able to do that.

Growing larger during this trimester meant dealing with some unpleasant changes too. First, my back began to bother me in ways it never had when I carried just one baby. My upper back would ache after a day of working, but it was my lower back that really hurt. I did everything to relieve that pain—ice packs, hot packs. My favorite was the heating pad, which I kept by my bed. I also had a chiropractor that was very good, and he figured out ways to adjust my back in spite of my big belly. I'd lie on my side, or I'd sit on a special chair and lean forward so he could work on me. This was when James started massaging me too, especially to loosen my shoulder muscles and ease the tension in my upper back. I've heard that there is even a certain type of massage table that comfortably and safely cradles a very pregnant belly. I didn't go to a masseuse who had one of those tables, but I'd highly recommend treating yourself to a massage of any kind as often as possible, done by a masseuse who is familiar with working on pregnant women, or by a helpful, willing husband.

Next to my husband and my heating pad, my best friends during this pregnancy were my pillows! I accumulated lots of them, in different sizes, so I could invent combinations that cushioned me wherever I most needed it. If there's one thing I'd recommend every pregnant woman get it's a large collection of pillows. Around my fifth month I started sleeping on my side with a pillow between my knees, which really helped my back. I still sleep that way. One friend told me she used a small pillow under her belly to prop it up as well. When I sat up in bed to read, a foam wedge beneath my knees took the strain off my back. I used various sizes of slanted pillows for my head, and I came to love my buckwheat pillows. A buckwheat pillow is heavier than the usual pillow, but you can mold it to fit where you want it. I liked having a lot of smaller pillows, but some of my friends swear by those huge body pillows. You'll have to experiment to see what's most comfortable for you, but if you have a good number of pillows in a wide variety of shapes and sizes, I know you'll find there is an infinite number of ways they'll help you get comfortable as you grow.

Unfortunately, the pillows didn't help with the leg cramps I started getting at night—another aspect of this pregnancy that was new to me. Oh, those cramps, they were terrible! I'd wake up completely panicked and screaming, "My leg! My leg!" It felt like my calf muscle was about to snap in two. James would immediately be there, massaging my leg, working the cramp out. He was just fabulous about that. If I had one during the day, he'd literally drop everything and come running, but they were much more common at night. When I mentioned them to Dr. Ross during a regular checkup, she said most pregnant women get them, and it signifies a shortage of calcium. She told me to take three additional Tums for more calcium. Still, I was enormously glad I had James by my side most of the time! He could make them go away if I straightened my leg and flexed my ankle while he gently massaged my calf muscle.

How You May Feel in Mid-Pregnancy

Most women find they still have many of the early pregnancy symptoms (except nausea) at this time. You might also experience:

- continually enlarging, and tender, breasts.
- occasional headaches, faintness, or dizziness, especially if you change position quickly.
- a very healthy appetite.
- nasal congestion, occasional nosebleeds, or bleeding gums because of increased blood volume.
- mood swings or a feeling of being scatterbrained.
- swelling ankles and feet as the uterus presses on veins, slowing the return of blood to the heart.
- shortness of breath as the uterus expands upward to crowd the lungs.
- difficulty sleeping as it becomes more difficult to find a comfortable position.

I'm not sure how much my growing belly had to do with the constipation I had from the second trimester on, because I've had this problem off and on all my life, but it definitely became a constant issue. Dr. Ross told me it might be made worse by the iron in my prenatal vitamins, or it could have been the fact that at this stage of pregnancy, all the internal organs are cramped for space. At the same time, she said that the muscles in the intestines are relaxed because of pregnancy hormones, so they don't move as well. In any case, she said most women could just drink more water and eat more fiber-rich foods, although constipation can be a persistent problem, especially in women pregnant with twins. Some women also need a stool softener too, before they see results. But since this was also a problem for me before I was pregnant, Dr. Ross told me to just keep using the over-the-counter product with psyllium seed I'd used anyway, and adjust the dose or the frequency to whatever I needed. That was a relief.

Your Checkups

By this time you might be feeling as if you're practically living at the doctor's office. I know I did. With all the monitoring, and the nurse on the set constantly checking my blood pressure, I never had a moment when I could forget I was pregnant. I was aware every minute of the day of the precious cargo I was carrying. For the most part that was fine. But I have to admit there were days that it got a little old by the middle of the second trimester. It seemed no one—myself included—had a single thought that didn't include babies or pregnancy. At times, when I'd be so weary of all the attention this pregnancy demanded I felt a little ungrateful. But I do believe that weariness was perfectly normal. Some evenings, mostly on the weekend when I wasn't too tired from working, James and I would stay home, cuddle up on the couch and watch a light-hearted movie together. It was a great two-hour escape from the intensity of not only our working life, but from our pregnant life!

Dr. Ross continued to monitor my blood pressure daily through the nurse on the set, and I visited her office every two or

Gestational Diabetes

In addition to the routine assessments your doctor performed during the first trimester, at about your sixth month she will also check for gestational diabetes. Women pregnant with twins and those who are over 30, overweight, or who have a family history of diabetes are the likeliest candidates. In some women who are pregnant with twins, increased levels of placental hormones can interfere with the normal action of insulin. When that happens, blood sugar levels skyrocket, bringing on a temporary form of diabetes. If it's not controlled, gestational diabetes can produce low blood sugar and other metabolic problems in the babies shortly after they are born.

Gestational diabetes disappears when the pregnancy is over, although 50 percent of women who had it will get diabetes later in life. During the pregnancy, it is usually controllable with a special diet and exercise. Your doctor may ask a dietitian and/or a physician who specializes in diabetes to prescribe one for you. Some women do also require insulin injections.

Signs that you may have gestational diabetes:

- Excessive thirst.
- Increased frequency and volume of urination.
- Fatigue.
- Recurrent vaginal yeast infections.
- A urine test that shows elevated glucose levels.

If your doctor thinks you may have gestational diabetes, she should then give you a *glucose challenge test*.

three weeks. During one of those visits Dr. Ross said that because twins so often arrive at least two or three weeks early, I could be more than halfway through the pregnancy! I knew perfectly well how far along I was, but still that came as kind of a shock. On the one hand, I had been feeling as though I'd been pregnant for most of my life. On the other it seemed too soon to be looking toward the end of the pregnancy. The effect of what she'd said was probably exactly what she'd hoped it would be—I realized time was flying by and I didn't have forever to make the most of this pregnancy for the babies. I immediately redoubled my efforts to gain weight, and I tried to cut my activity even more to be sure the babies stayed *in utero* for as long as possible. I was thrilled at our next visit to see that I'd gained a total of 31 pounds so far!

Several weeks later, when I was exactly 28 weeks pregnant in mid-October, we had just finished rehearsing a scene and I was standing under a tree, as I recall, waiting for the cameramen to be ready to film the scene, which was to be a close-up. Just as the director called, "Action!" a huge contraction gripped me. My eyes just went wide, I bent over and I instinctively started doing my Lamaze breathing. I remember being aware that the whole crew was just standing there looking at me, I assume wondering what in the world was going on. It was pretty frightening really. I was shocked at the idea I would be having contractions so early, and I was trying hard to be brave and not to alarm everyone. But I knew I was in trouble.

Having been pregnant before, I was familiar with both the "real" contractions of labor and with Braxton-Hicks contractions, the "practice" tensing and releasing of uterine muscles that begins in the second trimester. Several times a day I could feel the muscles across my belly bunch and tighten, then relax, and I wasn't alarmed by it. But this was different—it was much stronger than the usual Braxton-Hicks contraction, and lower. I felt tremendous pelvic pressure. I had James take me to Dr. Ross' office immediately. When she told me she wanted to do a few tests, just to be sure everything was all right, I'm sure my blood pressure went up several points, but I was glad to be in her care.

After hooking me up to an external monitor that fastened around my belly like a belt, Dr. Ross announced that what I had thought were contractions were what she called an "irritable uterus." She added that because my cervix had not changed, I was not in preterm labor. Thank goodness! But the whole episode frightened me. I was 28 weeks pregnant. My goal had been to make it to at least 34 weeks, longer if possible. I knew that if I did go into labor and the babies were born at 28 weeks, they would be called *very early preterm*. In that case, we could expect that they would not only be in the hospital for weeks or months, but that they stood a good chance of having long-term medical problems.

How Likely Is It for Twins to be Born Prematurely?

Approximately 50 percent of twins are born prematurely, or before the end of 37 weeks of pregnancy. By comparison, about 10 percent of singleton babies are premature, 90 percent of triplets and almost all quadruplets. Pre-term birth is the leading cause of neonatal death in the U.S., and among premature babies; one in ten do not survive. Those who do survive are at risk for a variety of medical problems. The earlier the birth, the higher the risk. Babies born earlier than 24 weeks are often not viable. Babies born from 25–28 weeks often survive (at 28 weeks about 90 percent survive) but they are at substantial risk for medical problems; from 29–32 weeks the outlook is pretty good, although the babies will likely be hospitalized for several weeks or more. Twins are often born between 33–35 weeks, and at this age they are not likely to spend a lot of time in the hospital or to have serious complications. Twins born between 36 and 38 weeks are considered full-term babies, and are generally as healthy as full-term singletons. They usually go home from the hospital when their mother is discharged.

After spending hours being monitored, I was so bored and so lonely I was quite certain I didn't want to have to be on bed rest for months. As if that wasn't enough motivation to be sure I didn't overdo, before I left her office that day, Dr. Ross had me go over to the hospital to visit the intensive care nursery where the premature babies were. They were so tiny and their parents looked so worried, watching their every breath; it really made an impression on me. I promised Dr. Ross I'd do what she told me to do in order to keep the babies inside for as long as possible, and to keep me off of total bed rest! Of course I would have gone to bed in an instant if she'd told me I needed to, but I didn't relish the thought, and I really wanted to do what was best for the babies and for me.

Warning Signs of Pre-Term Labor

Call your doctor *immediately* if you experience any one of these symptoms:

- Four or more contractions an hour.
- Rhythmic or persistent pelvic or lower abdominal pressure.
- Menstrual-like cramps, with or without diarrhea.
- Sudden or persistent low backache.
- Vaginal discharge, or a change in the type of vaginal discharge.
- Bleeding.
- A rush or steady trickle of fluid from the vagina.

While she was monitoring me, Dr. Ross also saw that I had an excess of amniotic fluid, a condition called *polyhydramnios*. It can be a sign of structural problems for the babies, but because of the frequent and detailed ultrasounds we'd had, we knew that wasn't the case. She did joke that having two out of the three most common complications of pregnancy for mothers of twins— contractions at 28 weeks (which I did not have), high blood pressure, and excess amniotic fluid—don't always all happen to the same person. We really hit the jackpot!

Before I went home, Dr. Ross spent time consulting with a perinatologist about how exactly they should handle the irritable uterus issue. She discussed it thoroughly with me, and assured me that if either she or the perinatologist thought for a minute that I had actually been in pre-term labor, I would not be going home at all. Still, they decided that one more preventive measure was a good idea. So, Dr. Ross sent me home with a terbutaline pump system that would inject me with the correct dose of the contraction-stopping medication if I started having contractions. If you've been given one of these, the likelihood is that you are (or will soon be) on bed rest because you have had pre-term labor. I can assure you, there won't be any walking around the house or going to work, even if you are putting your feet up! The pump itself is a small box that held both the medicine and the needle that injected the medicine at the correct intervals. I taped it to the front of one of my thighs, and then every three days, I had to move it to the other thigh. It wasn't a lot of fun, because I was re-injecting myself with each move, but at least the needle wasn't too long. Because the dosage depended on whether I was having contractions, I also had to monitor myself daily. I had a monitor at home, attached to a computer and once or twice a day I'd strap on the monitor belt and the readings would be sent to Dr. Ross over the telephone lines. I actually had to be quite together about numbers, figures, dials and buttons. James helped a lot, but there was plenty of opportunity to be confused by it all.

As another precaution, Dr. Ross also gave me instructions to lie down and rest as much as possible. Usually, she told me, she recommends that women pregnant with twins cut their activity by at least 50 percent by the time they've reached 28 weeks. But if a woman has been hospitalized for pre-term labor with cervical changes, she said it undoubtedly happens again, so the prescription is complete bed rest, close monitoring and drug therapy. Fortunately, I hadn't had pre-term labor, just an extremely irritable uterus. Consequently, my prescription to reduce my activity, monitor myself, and to use the terbutaline pump was purely preventative.

What Causes Pre-Term Labor?

Sometimes it's a mystery, but there are some things we know can trigger contractions and even cervical changes long before the due date:

- Carrying multiples.
- Polyhydramnios.
- Vaginal infections.
- Urinary tract infections.
- A cervix that has been weakened or damaged.
- Placenta previa in which the placenta covers the cervix, or placental abruption in which the placenta comes away from the uterine wall.
- Structural malformation, or failure to thrive of either or both babies.
- Mother's medical condition such as long-standing (not gestational) diabetes, or high blood pressure.
- Mother's inadequate nutrition.
- Exposure to alcohol, cigarettes or recreational drugs.
- Spontaneous rupture of membranes.

Because of our shooting schedule on *Dr. Quinn,* I couldn't stay home yet but I was determined to adjust my working environment to my babies' needs. I usually had a driver who took me to the set, but thank goodness for Jana Riportella, who was willing to do more than just drive me here and there. She was a good friend of Patrice who had come up with the idea for matzoh ball soup when I had been so sick. The two of them worked together to be sure I was as inactive as possible. One morning, after driving me to the set, Jana hauled from the trunk of the car a huge chaise lounge-style, portable garden chair, which she carried to my trailer. On the set—and in my personal life—my routine was intimately involved with that chair. When we were shooting a scene, I'd carefully lie down on it (with help) and watch the young woman who had been hired to stand in for me as she and the other actors rehearsed. When all was ready, I'd very carefully get up (with help), Kelly and Lesa would check my hair and makeup, and I'd perform my part. Then it was back to the chaise for me. That was my version of "bed rest" in the middle of *Dr. Quinn, Medicine Woman*—with the dust, the dirt, the heat, the horses, and the rattlesnakes!

What Can Be Done to Stop Labor?

Several medications, called *tocolytics,* are typically used to stop or slow labor. They are terbutaline, indomethacin, isoxsupine and ritodrine.

While studies have shown that no major abnormalities have been reported in newborns treated with tocolytics while in utero, there are often side effects that can be uncomfortable for the mother. Some possible side effects of tocolytics for the mother are: palpitations or rapid pulse, tremors, dizziness, nausea/vomiting, nervousness/restlessness, sleeplessness, depression, hot flashes/heat intolerance, chest pains or tightness, ringing in the ears, shortness of breath, rashes, constipation or diarrhea, bloating.

Another medication used to slow labor, which isn't technically a tocolytic, is magnesium sulfate.

Your Babies, As They Grow

At every visit I had with Dr. Ross, she continued to check on how the babies were growing. We'd known for a time that they were fraternal boys and with ultrasounds done every three weeks, James and I felt like we were really getting to know them. We could actually see them develop.

How Your Babies Grow During Mid-Pregnancy

Weeks 16–20: This is a big growth period, and by the end of it each baby is about seven and a half inches long. By now they have developed a sense of taste and they respond to bright lights outside the mother's body. Ultrasounds show twins kicking and jostling each other at this point.

Weeks 20–24: Babies often fall asleep while mom is walking around, and wake up when she is quiet. When they are awake, they are liable to be constantly kicking you and each other. They weigh about a pound each. By about 20 weeks most women can feel their babies moving.

Weeks 24–28: The babies continue to develop their own individual cycles of sleeping and waking, cycles that will continue after their births. By 28 weeks your twins may weigh as much as three pounds each and be as much as 15 inches long.

I'd been able to feel the babies moving since sometime during the fourth month. I don't remember a specific moment when I felt them moving for the first time. In previous pregnancies, when I'd had only one baby at a time, I did have a definite moment when I thought,

"Aha! That's a baby kicking." As those pregnancies went on, I could feel a whole arm or a leg surface as the baby rolled around.

With twins however, it seemed there was just a lot of movement in general, and I felt it pretty early on. But I never could distinguish an arm or a leg. What I could distinguish was a difference in the amount of movement between the two babies. The one who spent most of the time on the right side I could always feel kicking and moving. The one on the left kicked a bit, but was nowhere near as active as the one on the right. They seemed to stay in the same places for the most part—which makes sense because there just wasn't that much room in there. We could of course identify who was where through the ultrasounds, and sure enough, the one on the right was Kris, our active boy, and the one on the left was John, head down, quietly waiting to get out.

As the boys grew, I still felt movement, but it became less and less dramatic as they ran out of room. I pictured them being a bit crushed in there, but they managed to wiggle plenty, let me assure you!

What's Special About the 20-Week Ultrasound?

During the second trimester, your doctor should evaluate your babies' growth rate by ultrasound to be sure each is getting a fair share of placental nutrients. Genetic differences that may one day make one taller than the other will not have shown up yet, so they should be close to the same size—some doctors say within 20 percent of each other in size and weight.

If there is a large size discrepancy, your doctor will probably want to follow you closely to see if the smaller baby catches up and to be sure your nutrition is more than adequate. Later in the pregnancy, in some cases when one baby stops growing, both babies are delivered to ensure the health of the smaller one.

Your Self, Your Family

Inactivity is a foreign concept to me. The idea of sitting still and not doing anything is just not part of my makeup. Even though I was ready and willing to slow down after my scare over possible pre-term labor, it was still very difficult—as I think it is for most women. Whether we are home with small children or the mainstay at the office, most of us today shoulder a good deal of responsibility in one way or another. Figuring out how to deal with that and do what's best for our babies is not always easy.

Painting continued to be my passion and my path toward peacefulness. It was one thing I could do without running around that I really enjoyed. So that's what I happily did. Two or three of my favorite paintings came out of that period. But at the same time, the painting that was on my mind every day was of a different sort— that of the babies' room. We had decided to turn a guestroom off the living room into a nursery. It was just steps away from our bedroom, so the location was ideal. But we couldn't decide on colors or a decorating theme for the longest time, and I'd begun to think we'd just paint it blue, or something simple like that.

Meanwhile, friends and fans continued to send gifts for the babies; it seemed we were getting something every day. And those gifts were what finally gave me the idea for the boys' room. By the end of my second trimester, we'd received more than a dozen sets of stuffed animals. Because I was having twins, we were being given two teddy bears, two giraffes, two monkeys, two of everything. Opening yet another box, this one with two little gorillas, I had a revelation: why not do the boys' room with a jungle theme, and use the dozens of stuffed animals as part of that theme! James, Katie, Sean and I all played around with that idea for a while, and I came up with the brilliant notion that we could use cup hooks to hang the animals, two by two, on the walls. So today the boys sleep beneath a glorious painted mural of rain forest trees and vines, as stuffed monkeys and teddy bears swing two by two through the branches.

As it turned out, planning and painting the boys' room, and sorting all those toys, became a wonderful family project. Katie and Sean liked the idea of getting ready for the babies, and they especially liked the fact that some of their own creativity went into getting the babies' room ready.

The Straight Scoop: Notes for Dads from James

By the middle of her pregnancy, Jane was not only working hard at finishing the episodes for *Dr. Quinn*; she was also working hard at taking care of herself and the babies. That wasn't always easy for her, I could see that. At first, I felt a little helpless—what could I do that wasn't just nagging her to eat more and exercise carefully?

When the answer finally hit me, I thought it was brilliant. I would go into training with her, become part of what she was doing. I actually did improve my eating habits and exercise more, so we were doing this together, and I think she appreciated the company, as well as the empathy. But we did say that probably not all guys should eat the way a woman pregnant with twins ate, or they'd have matching bellies!

Seriously, I did take the approach that I would use this time to be in the best shape of my life when the babies were born, in every way. On more than just the physical level, I felt that I was in training to be the best father I could be.

Looking Good, Feeling Good

Let's face it. As those of us who are having twins get farther along in our pregnancies, the idea of looking really good has to be seriously adjusted. By the middle of our pregnancies, many of us will have bellies as large as those of a woman ready to deliver—and theoretically we have nearly three months left to go! There were days when I was astounded at my size. Stepping out of the shower, I'd stand sideways before the mirror in awe, and I'd think this must be the biggest my belly could be. But the next week, I'd do the same thing again. One friend told me that while she was pregnant with twins she had the distinct sensation on some days that she could actually feel her great belly expanding, growing even larger!

One of the adjustments I made in the way I dressed was to put the visual emphasis somewhere besides on my belly, if it was at all possible. Also, I had come to see the huge mound that dominated my body as something glorious. Whenever I thought of the two boys jostling and kicking inside, I had no problem adjusting my attitude. It was truly a glorious sight.

Exercise

Before I say anything at all about exercising during mid-pregnancy, I want to repeat myself about being sure it is right for you to exercise now. *You should absolutely not exercise if your doctor has told you not to, if you have a history of miscarriage, or if for any reason you think you are likely to—or have already—experienced even the most minor signs of pre-term labor!* The best place for your babies is in the womb, and everything you do must support them staying there for as long as they can.

That said, there are exercises you can do to maintain some level of fitness during your pregnancy. Dr. Ross approved every exercise I did first. If you do work out, or if you find a trainer who specializes in pregnancy workouts, I suggest you do the same. Have *every* exercise approved by your doctor before you move a muscle.

The trainer I worked with, Birgitta Gallo noticed that the larger my belly grew, the more my aching lower back was arching, and the more my shoulders were rounding. The workout she designed for me focused on strengthening those areas as well as the muscles supporting the hips. Joints naturally loosen during pregnancy, as a result of the hormones that prepare your body to give birth. Birgitta told me that's why many women have that waddling look when they walk—because of loose hip joints and a lessening of tone in the surrounding muscles. But I have to say that by the end of a pregnancy, especially a twin pregnancy, I don't think any woman walks like she did before she was pregnant, no matter how much she has exercised. There's simply too much in the way!

We also did some childbirth preparation exercises like Kegels, which I had already started in the first trimester, and the C-Curve, which stretches the lower back and buttocks by curving the body forward in the shape of a letter C. (See illustration.) And we did exercises for the abdominal muscles to keep them toned and supple, both for the birth and to make getting back my pre-twins shape a little easier after the birth. The workout also allowed me to keep my arms and legs in shape.

Birgitta tried to vary the specific exercises I would do so that it wouldn't be too boring. We worked out three times a week, and before I was on the terbutaline pump, we alternated gym work-

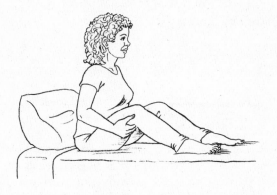

Sit up straight in bed with your knees bent, holding them from behind for support. Round your back, pull your abdomen in and hold for 10–30 seconds. Repeat.

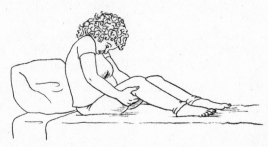

outs with pool workouts, where I did essentially the same exercises using the water or I used special pool exercise tools for resistance. In fact, if there is a pool available to you, water workouts may be the best and safest way for you to exercise. It was so soothing to be in the water and not to feel all the extra weight I carried for a while. That in itself was relaxing!

My workout is a good one for any woman pregnant with twins who has exercised a bit already. If you'd like to use it, be sure your doctor approves, or makes modifications that fit your needs.

Every Woman's Twin-Pregnancy Workout

Warm-up: 10–20 minutes on the StairMaster or the recumbent bike. (But as soon as I had the irritable uterus episode, all cardiovascular warm-ups were out!)

Upper back/Neck: Lat Pulldowns (on a weight machine or using stretchy bands)

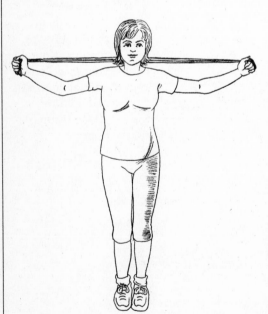

Stand or sit straight, pulling in your abdominal muscles. With a stretchy exercise band wrapped around your fingers, reach with your arms in a V shape over your head. Open your arms slowly, pull the band down behind your neck, squeezing your shoulder blades together.

Rear Shoulder Pull (using stretchy exercise bands)
Scapular Retraction (using dumbbells)

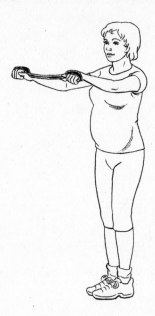

Hold the exercise band in front of you at chest height, hands shoulder-width apart. Press your arms apart and backward using your rear shoulder muscles. Return to starting position and repeat.

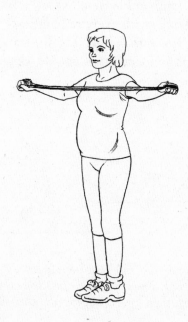

Lower back/ Kneeling Pelvic Tilt with Kegels
Abdominals: Dog Wag (wagging hips, on hands and knees)
Seated Crunches (on physio ball or chair—see illustration)

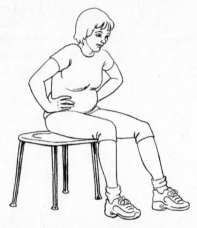

Sitting down, contract stomach muscles downward, exhaling as you contract. Inhale as you release.

Legs: Side Leg Lifts (with ankle weights) or
Sideways Walking (with exercise bands)
Supported Squats with Kegels (see illustration)
Leg Extensions and Curls (with ankle weights)

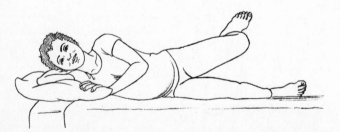

Lying on your right side, bend your right leg for support. With left leg straight and foot flexed, slowly bend at the knee and raise the leg about 12 inches, then lower. Repeat on other side.

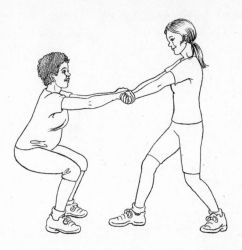

Stand with your feet shoulder-width apart. Holding on to something sturdy, such as a person or a heavy piece of furniture, squat down as far as is comfortable. Be sure to keep your back straight with your abdominals pulled in and your knees behind your toes. Press up using your thighs, feeling the pressure through your heels. If this bothers your knees or your back, this exercise is not right for you.

Chest and Arms:	Chest Press or Flyes (on Pilates machine)
	Seated Biceps Curls (with dumbbells)
	Triceps Pushdown (on weight machine)

Childbirth	C-Curve
Prep:	Hip Openers (see illustration)
	Kegels

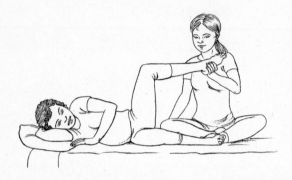

Lie on your right side, both legs bent. Lift the left knee until it is perpendicular to the bed. Slowly release. Repeat on the other side.

Cool Down: Gentle Stretching

Note: You'll find a workout modified for those on bed rest on page 104.

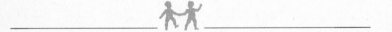

My workout was a regular part of my schedule, but there were days that shooting kept me from being home to meet Birgitta. On those days, I did what I could on the set. I must have looked a bizarre sight hiking up my 19th century skirts so I could do my sideways walking exercises with stretchy exercise bands around my ankles!

Dressing Well

For most of this trimester, we were still hiding my pregnancy on the show. Keeping the same general silhouette, as we did in the first trimester, was out of the question now, so they hid me behind candles or flowers, or had me seated at a table. I couldn't always be hidden though, so I also started wearing a long canvas coat called a duster, which was of the period, and it conveniently hid not only my growing middle, but also my entire body.

Near the end of my second trimester, the story line had caught up with us, and Michaela was pregnant at last. Finally, my own pregnancy could show. Cheri had been researching 19th century maternity clothing as the first step in designing some pieces for me on the show. But there was a catch, she soon found. Women at that time didn't have their pictures made when they were pregnant, and they really didn't go out of the house much during their pregnancies—we've all heard the term "confinement." So she had trouble at first even finding pictures of period clothing for pregnant women. When she did we were all shocked to find that women then still wore corsets early in their pregnancies, and they put themselves right back into their corsets immediately afterward! When India rubber began to be used in clothing in the early 19th century, they did put some in the corsets, so they'd stretch a little, but all in all, it sounded pretty uncomfortable to me.

I never wore corsets on the show, I can assure you. But I did really like some of the things Cheri designed for me. Long skirts with a shirt worn on the outside, or wrapper dresses were really quite comfortable. I also liked the empire-style dresses with the high waist, lightly gathered under the bust.

While I had no interest in wearing a corset, and I'm sure no one would recommend any pregnant woman would wear one, I did feel I needed some support for my belly, and the loose skirts and dresses couldn't provide that. In my personal life, I'd taken to wearing spandex shorts, like bicycle shorts without the seat padding, under some of my dresses because they were comfortable and I felt the support helped my back as well as my belly. Cheri also noticed that when I was just standing around, my arms naturally ended up cradling my belly. You may have noticed that too—lightly clasping your hands beneath your belly does feel comfortable, maybe because there's no place else to put your hands! After all, there are a limited number of choices of what to do with them: they hang at your sides, you rest them on top of your belly, or they cradle your belly.

At any rate, Cheri noticed me cradling mine, she knew about my back problems, and those two facts gave her an idea. She created a combination of maternity underwear and tights for me that were heavenly to wear. Starting with a pair of spandex shorts, she added a large fabric flap made of stretchy cotton Lycra that went across the lower part of my belly and was held in place at the side by Velcro. I could adjust it as I grew and it really helped me feel supported on all sides. At the time, Cheri considered producing it commercially, which was a great idea, but other projects and her own pregnancy got in the way. Since then, I have noticed something similar on the market, which shouldn't be difficult to track down at a maternity store.

I was lucky that Cheri was also able to make clothing for my personal life. She used many of the same principles there that she used in creating costumes for the show, and I hope you'll find them useful in building your own maternity wardrobe. First of all, the type of fabric you wear becomes much more important when you're pregnant than at any other time. Cheri used fabrics with enough drape and weight that they'd fall softly and not cling to the body or to other fabrics. We always made sure everything was large enough in the seat to avoid any clinging. And our cardinal rule was that if two fabrics came into contact anywhere, a shirt worn out over pants for example, *they absolutely must be able to slide over each other and not catch or cling.* No one needs to have her backside silhouetted when she is pregnant! That's why we stayed away from 100 percent cotton tops or cotton pants. Instead, Cheri used a lot of polyester blends, often with Lycra so they'd have a bit of give to them. Crisp fabrics were also out. I don't wear them a lot in my personal life anyway, and we found that they only look good if they fall perfectly straight. If they touch any part of your body they look dumpy. And sometimes, they have to be so large to fall straight that they can end up making you look bigger than you are.

Cheri made several great looking dresses for me similar to the baby-doll dresses popular at the time. She used small, often monochromatic prints to minimize overall size. The colors were bright but not shocking; enough to perk me up on tired days, but not enough to make me look like a billboard. The dresses usually featured a flattering scooped neck, short sleeves and a slightly higher than normal waist. She was careful not to make the waist tight under the bust, but a little looser there to minimize breasts that had grown so large they were beginning to look a little out of control, especially on my short frame. I wore the spandex bike shorts or tights under the dresses, so I was very comfortable. Some days I added a broad-brimmed straw hat or perhaps a lovely scarf; each shifted the focus upward from the middle of the body. I have to say I always felt feminine and pretty in Cheri's creations.

If you are working in an office during your pregnancy, more tailored lines and crisper fabrics may be just the thing for you. In fact, a tailored jacket and a shirt with some body to it, worn outside trousers can look very slimming.

One last note: some of my friends who have had their babies one at a time look fabulous in clothing that outlines or somehow highlights their pregnant bellies. I remember a party where I saw one quite obviously pregnant friend in a velvet stretch catsuit, and she looked elegant. However, those of us who are pregnant with twins usually have bellies of an entirely different magnitude than those who are pregnant with one baby. Revealing, belly-defining outfits were not a look I favored.

Even so, just past the middle of my pregnancy, although I was wearing one of my most belly-minimizing dresses, a waiter, assuming I must be about to give birth at any time, assured me someone at the restaurant could take me to the hospital at a moment's notice!

Several months later when Cheri was pregnant herself, in her search for professional-looking clothing that fit, she began to shop in the plus-size department at her favorite stores rather than in the more expensive maternity shops. She could always find something fashionable, and bought only the pieces that would work for her. Like all of us, she wasn't enormously larger everywhere on her body, so certain pieces worked better than others did. One I remember was a chiffon shirt she could wear over a shell, and it always looked pretty and professional. Cheri also picked up some great stretch pants at boutique stores that worked for at least part of her pregnancy.

Cheri and I agreed that a few pieces of maternity clothing are essential, although they may vary depending on your lifestyle and what time of year you're pregnant. First, there's really no substitute for a good maternity bathing suit. Maternity jeans make a great basic for many women, and maternity pantyhose or tights are a must if you're pregnant with twins and need to dress up. I could get away with a larger size of regular hose in my other pregnancies, but not with twins.

Details

By the middle of your pregnancy, you may feel just like I did—that you need a bit of pampering. I certainly felt I deserved it! By now you probably have luxuriously thick hair and your skin is glowing, so I hope you're having fun with those plusses.

Another plus you might have noticed is that your nails are likely to be the best you've seen them. The same process that grows that thick pregnancy hair also grows long, lovely fingernails. Even if they're not long, my guess is they are strong. Take advantage and treat yourself to a manicure. I don't mind doing my own manicures, and often do these days, but I feel very pampered if someone else does it for me. While you're at it, I highly recommend a pedicure. If you haven't ever had one, trust me, it's the ultimate in relaxation. You probably can't reach your toes now anyway, and your feet may be feeling unusually tired as you grow—it's the perfect time to give them some attention.

If cost is a consideration, check with a local beauty school where students are likely to give manicures and pedicures for a very low fee. If friends have been asking you what they can do for you, tell them you're accepting checks in your Self-care Fund. Or, you could ask a friend to do one for you, or even request a gift certificate for a manicure and pedicure at the local spa—where they are likely to include a foot massage along with the nail polish.

Congratulations! You've made it through the middle of your pregnancy. After all this time, it's now only a matter of weeks until your babies will be here. These are important final weeks, during which your babies' lungs are maturing and they are gaining weight that will help them regulate their body temperatures after they are born. Now is the time for you to slow down and help ensure these developments happen for your babies *before* they are born. It won't be long now before you'll meet them both!

Checklist for Mid-Pregnancy

Begin:

- Slowing down, or cutting out activities you don't really need to be involved in.
- Taking childbirth preparation classes, if you haven't already done so.
- Planning for delivery. If you haven't already done so, take a tour of the hospital where you plan to deliver.
- Paying even closer attention to your body. Let your doctor know about any changes you detect, no matter how small.
- Arranging for care for your other children. You need time to rest now, and will need more in the near future. If you have more than one child, child care can allow you to spend quiet time alone with each, reading or playing quiet games.
- Allowing your husband or friends to do part of what you normally do. Someone else can throw in a load of laundry while you rest. Ask friends who want to help to bring over one or two meals a week, or to run to the grocery store for you.

Put Off:

- Any major travel. You don't need the stress right now.
- Projects at work, which require extra energy or effort.
- Getting involved in volunteer work that will require you to do more than make a few telephone calls.

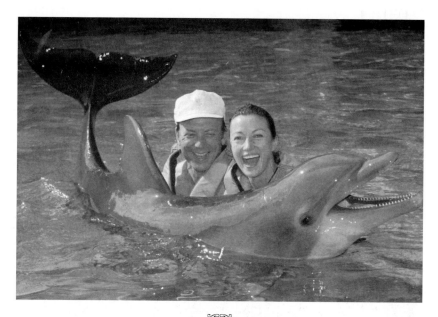

James and I swimming with dolphins for luck. Waiting to hear whether or not we are pregnant! (Author collection)

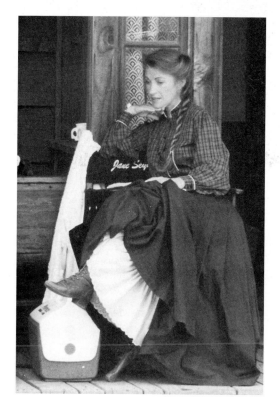

Taking a break on the set with my cooler of nutritious snacks nearby. (Andrea Daoutis)

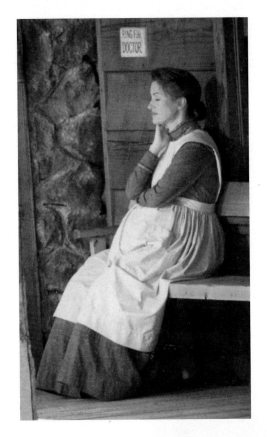

I tried to take catnaps on the set as often as possible, trying to conserve what little energy I had left.
(Andrea Daoutis)

At work on the set.
(Andrea Daoutis)

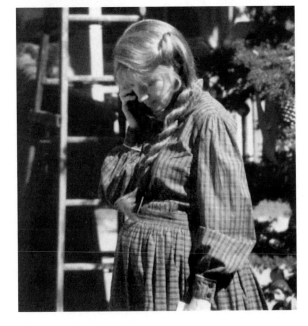

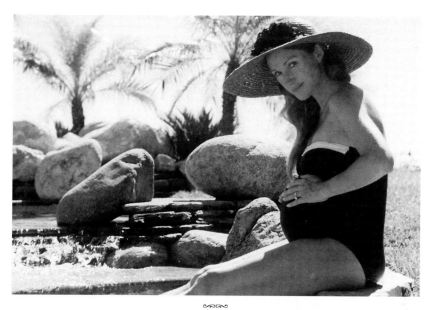

Just about halfway through my pregnancy. (Author collection)

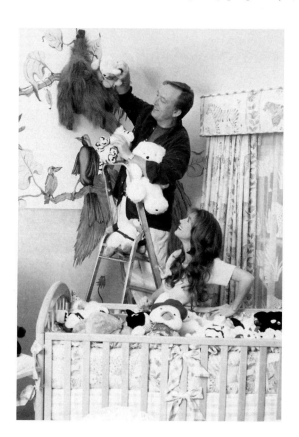

Decorating the nursery with two of everything. We used cup hooks to hang the stuffed animals on the mural. (Charles Bush)

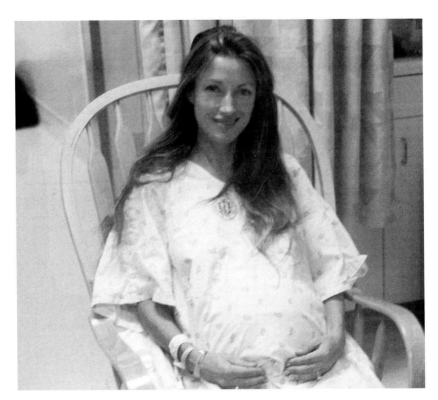

Any minute now! (Author collection)

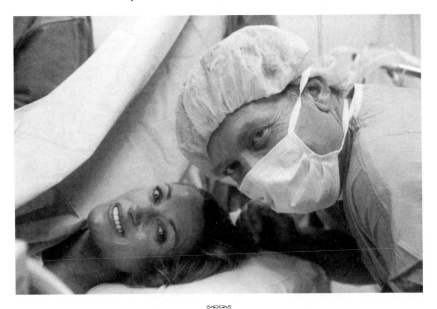

Waiting to deliver. (Author collection)

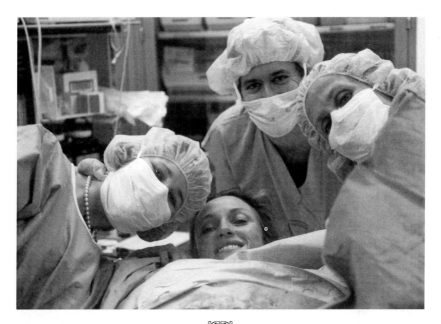

My team. (Author collection)

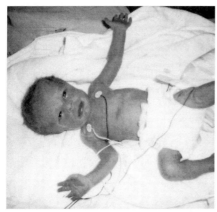

One hour old. John Stacy Keach *(left)*, Kristopher Steven Keach *(below)*. (Author collection)

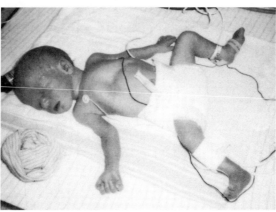

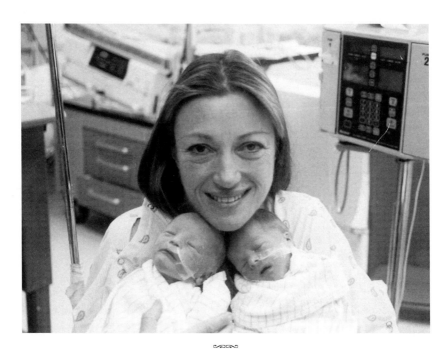

Exhausted but radiant with my two baby boys. (Author collection)

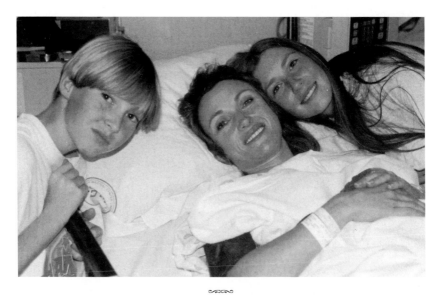

With Katie and Sean after delivery. (Author collection)

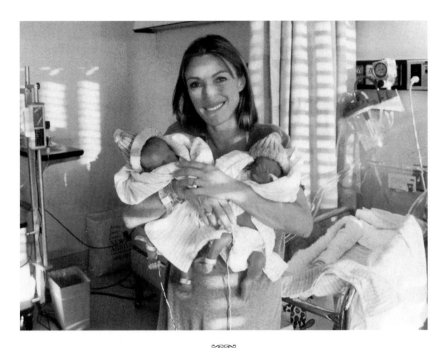

Feeling better now, but still in the NICU. (Author collection)

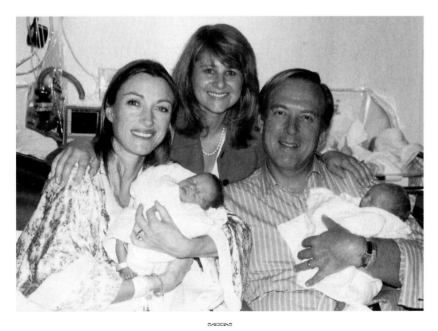

James, the boys and I with Dr. Sheryl Ross. (Author collection)

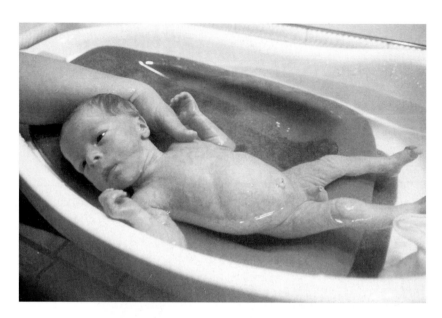

First baths! (Author collection)

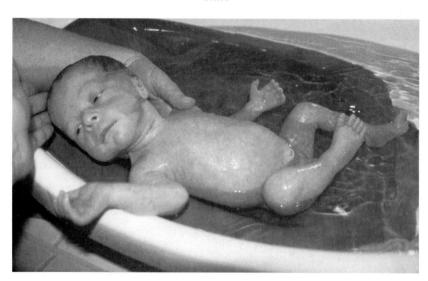

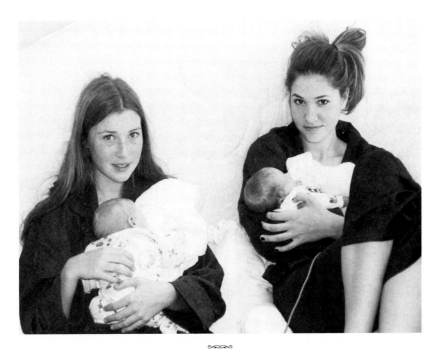

Katie *(left)* and Jenni *(right)* at home with the boys.
(Author collection)

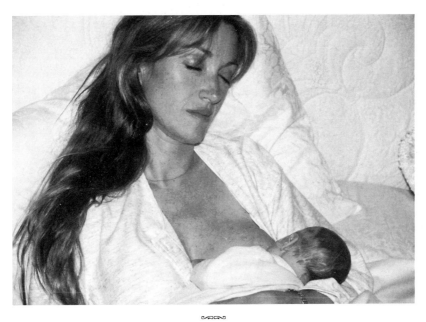

Having a nap while breast feeding. (Author collection)

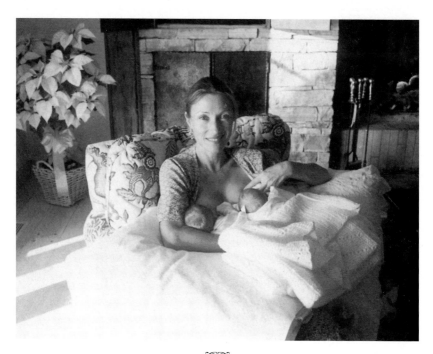

Breast feeding—TWO AT A TIME! (Author collection)

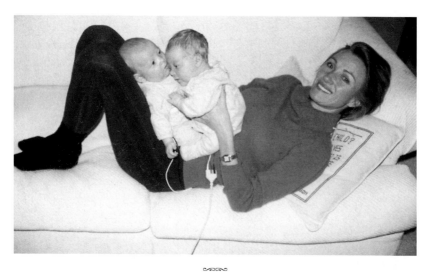

Three weeks old. Still attached to their monitors.
(Author collection)

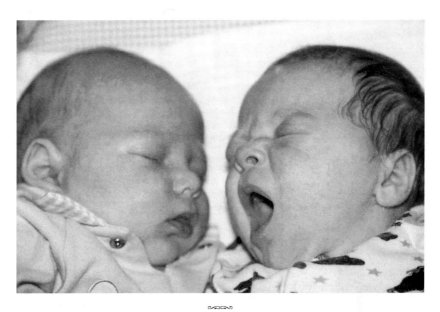

Kris and John, snuggling in their shared bassinet. (Author collection)

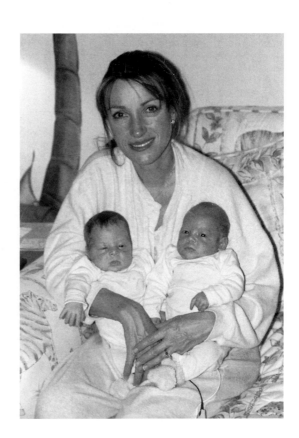

At home in
the nursery.
(Author collection)

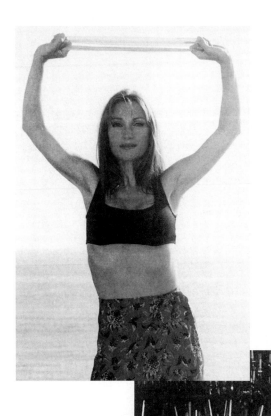

The exercise routines
worked! Six weeks
postpartum.
(Author collection)

The dress I wore to
the Golden Globe
Awards. Six weeks
postpartum!
(Author collection)

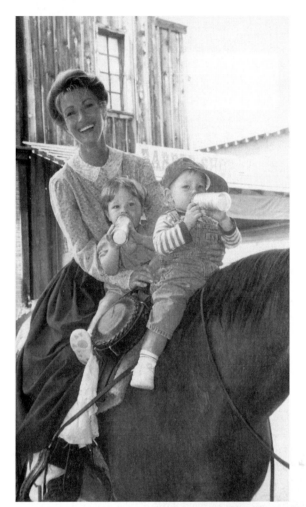

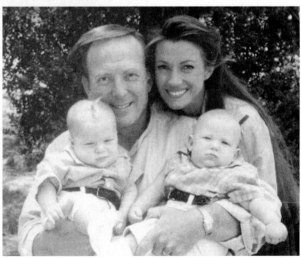

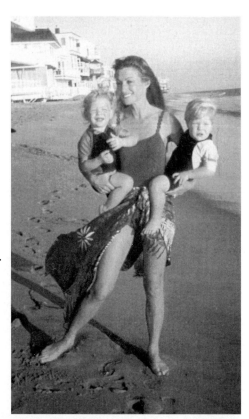

On the beach near our home.
(Author collection)

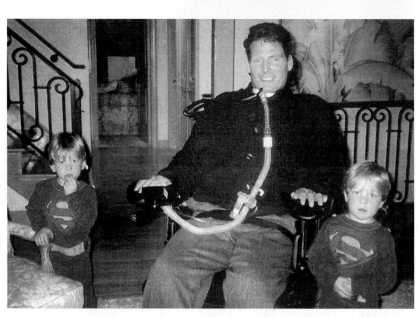

Supermen! Kris and John with my good friend
Christopher Reeve. (Author collection)

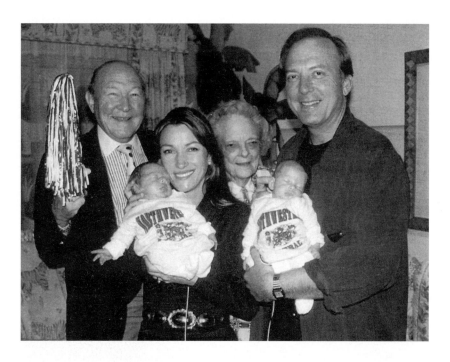

James, the boys and I with his parents *(above)* and with their grandmothers in their christening gowns *(below)*. (Author collection)

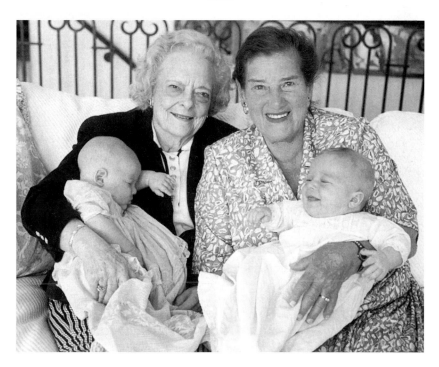

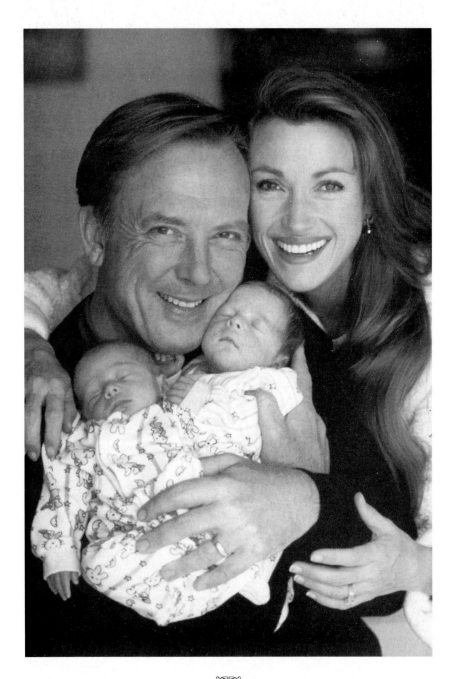

A favorite family photo. (Charles Bush)

four

Coming into the
Homestretch

Weeks 29–Birth

Watching and waiting. That's what my pregnancy was all about from the time I hit 29 weeks near the end of October until the boys were born. During these final weeks, I was very conscious of just waiting for it to be over. I definitely wanted my babies to stay inside for as long as they needed to, I really did. But still, I kept hearing this little voice in my head, repeating a single phrase: "Are we there yet?"

I know my doctor would describe these weeks differently. She kept reminding me that the last weeks of a twin pregnancy is where all the action is. The possibility of pre-term labor is always there, and she reminded me that anything short of the end of the 36th week was pre-term. So I was constantly on the lookout for signs that labor might start—too soon.

Believe it or not, the terbutaline pump became a real bright spot for me. I wore it every day, taped to my thigh beneath the stretchy tights I wore at home and the 19th century skirts I wore on the set. Even though it meant I had one more needle to contend with, I came to think the pump system was brilliant. While nothing could be an absolute guarantee that contractions wouldn't start before we wanted them to, knowing that I was constantly getting the right dose of medication to keep them away gave me a lot of comfort. That little pump was like a talisman of 20th century medicine that Michaela Quinn could only have dreamed about, if she'd imagined it at all.

In addition to wearing the pump, we continued with the other precautions. The nurse who was on the set anyway took my blood pressure several times a day, and James and I strapped on the monitor belt at home at least twice a day to check for contractions. When I wasn't being checked and monitored, I spent the greater part of my days on the set lying on the garden chaise, watching my stand-in rehearse while I went over my lines in my head.

Another bright spot was that I was finally *playing* pregnant on *Dr. Quinn* as well as *being* pregnant in real life. That was a lot easier than hiding the pregnancy on the show although the end result was that I had the longest human "pregnancy" the world had ever seen. In all, for *two years* I was either pregnant and hiding it on the show, pregnant and playing it on the show, or later, after the boys were born, not pregnant any more, but still playing pregnant on the show!

Your Pregnant Body

After my experience with the irritable uterus, everyone on the set as well as James and I knew that even if we could keep labor at bay until closer to my due date, my time was drawing near. So we did everything we could to achieve two important goals: take care of the babies, and get more episodes done before the babies were born. We started doing what we call in the business "bookends." I'd appear in only the beginning and the ending of an episode, and we'd shoot only my parts and no one else's. Instead of shooting one episode in seven days, as we usually did, we shot three episodes of my work alone in those seven days. It was very hard on everyone, although it was good for the series because it meant I (or rather, Michaela Quinn) could appear in every episode, as usual. However it also meant the writers had to write the shows farther in advance than they were used to, and it was tough for the other actors because we were working in such a piecemeal fashion. On the other hand, the crew and other actors were able to shoot for at least another three weeks after I left. And, once we'd finished those episodes, I knew I could leave work, confident that I'd done my job both for the babies and for the show.

Now that you've reached this last part of your pregnancy, perhaps you're feeling the same way. I hope you've already cut your activity by about 50 percent (it's best if you do that by 20 to 28 weeks), so you should be able to just continue gearing down. If you're still working outside the home, it is time to start wrapping up details and preparing in a more real way for the babies. If you're home already, (or on bed rest, which I'll talk about later in this chapter), you have the comfort of knowing you're almost there! Remember—twins are typically born at about 36 to 38 weeks, so there really isn't much time left in this pregnancy.

And it's a good thing, you might be saying to yourself, as I was at this point. How much bigger can I be? When I asked her this question, Dr. Ross reminded me that it was all for a good cause. This is the time when the babies continue to put on weight (although twins are usually gaining at a slower rate at this point in your pregnancy), adding the fat that will help them to regulate their body temperatures after they are born. So yes, she said, your belly should continue to grow during these last weeks, impossible as that may sound. If it's any comfort to you, Cheri, who measured me constantly for costumes she made, tells me I went from having a 24-inch waist before I was pregnant to—just before the boys were born—measuring 54 inches around my belly where my waist used to be!

In fact, it was around this time that my favorite "big belly" story happened, when I had just finished shooting *Dr. Quinn*. Time had passed since my uterus was "irritable," and it had seemed to calm down, so Dr. Ross agreed to let me attend one of my son Sean's soccer games at the field just down the street from our house. I went to his games as often as I could, but I certainly missed some because of my shooting schedule. Now that I was home, it was the perfect opportunity to catch up on my soccer game attendance, so long as Dr. Ross approved. So down the street I went, James driving me, with my trusty chaise lounge lawn chair. I reclined next to the field and was enjoying the game when I noticed a young child staring at me. Suddenly, he was at my side, and just as suddenly he put his little hands on my very large boobs and then my huge belly, and yelled to his mom, "Mommy, what are these?"

His mother rushed over, apologizing and obviously embarrassed, but I could only laugh. "It's all just so *out there,* isn't it?" I said. "Who could blame him for being curious?"

In these last weeks of the pregnancy, the energy I'd felt earlier began to wane. I think it was just increasingly difficult to haul myself—and my belly—around. Only a few weeks earlier, the idea of bed rest had horrified me. But now, while I wasn't prepared to immobilize myself if I didn't have to, I did find that I needed—and took—more catnaps, and I definitely felt I was slowing down.

Catnaps were great, and increasingly I found I needed them to make up for the sleep I wasn't getting at night. Sleeping soundly all night was quickly becoming a distant memory. My pillows, which I'd always loved and which had really helped to make me comfortable, were an absolute necessity now. From my previous pregnancies, I knew that this pattern of sleeping only in bits and pieces was one way Mother Nature seemed to prepare us for having a new baby—or babies.

James and I checked with Dr. Ross and we began to look ahead, to choose which would be my last day of work. About a week before that day came, when I was just about 30 weeks pregnant, we had just finished shooting for the morning. I'd come into what was our lunch area, which was sort of a very drafty tent-like arrangement of benches and trestle tables where the crew always ate, with the wind and the rain blowing in some days. This was a lovely, sunny late fall day though, and when I walked in I saw someone had decorated the whole tent and all the tables incredibly with balloons and big ribbons everywhere. There was a huge stage area at one end, which was covered, completely covered, with huge beautifully wrapped gifts. The entire crew and cast were there, waiting for me. It was a huge surprise, an absolute shock to me. I just started crying; I couldn't believe it. It's embarrassing enough to have gifts at all, but everything here was in twos—two high chairs, two bassinets, two of everything, great mounds of double gifts. There must have been at least two hundred people there. One of the immediately useful gifts they gave me was a very comfortable rocking chair. I sat in the rocker and

---

How Can I Expect to Feel Late in My Pregnancy?

In a word, you're likely to feel *more* of everything. The size of your uterus at about 28–29 weeks will probably be the same or greater than that of a woman who is at term with a single baby. Your breasts will continue to grow, and you may need a larger and/or more supportive bra. If you've had trouble with hemorrhoids in previous pregnancies, or even if you've never had them before, hemorrhoids may start to be a problem because of the increased weight of the babies and the pressure they exert on your body. Growing babies may also mean that you feel particularly breathless, as they press upward on your diaphragm.

---

opened gifts, forever it seemed. We were given everything—*two* of everything I should say—that we could possibly need, including two darling toy boxes with a beautiful animal motif. People whom I barely knew on the crew, gave me lovely traditional sweater ensembles their mothers or aunts had knitted for me. I was quite taken aback by everyone's heartfelt generosity.

I remembered well that this kind of generosity doesn't always come pouring out when one is pregnant, and I think because of that I cherished this all the more. I had gotten quite a different reception when I was pregnant with Katie and acting in the Broadway play *Amadeus*. I was fired almost immediately after everyone knew I was pregnant! So by the time I would have been the guest of honor at a lovely baby shower, I was unemployed and living with my husband in California, wondering where I was going to get all the baby equipment I needed. I was given some items by my parents and friends, and I managed to borrow other things, but I did have to become rather resourceful. If you're concerned about collecting all you'll need for your babies, or even not sure of exactly what you will need, look ahead to Chapter 7 where I'll give you my thoughts on what's important and what's not in the world of twin baby gear.

After all the presents and food, including a lovely delicious cake, we went back to work to finish our shooting! Within a week, we completed my part of the season's episodes, and I could stop working. It was a huge relief. I did however go back to the set one day to say goodbye. James was still shooting—he was directing an episode—and I dropped by unexpectedly to officially say farewell to the cast and crew. It was a wonderful day—exciting really, more so than I had anticipated. Everyone was excited to see me, I was excited to see them but also very excited not to be working any more. So I was very casual. I thought I'd just say Hello and Goodbye to everyone and that would be it. But there was this incredible atmosphere of caring coming from the cast and crew I really hadn't expected. It's one thing when you and your husband and family are thrilled about having a baby. It's something else when your whole world, everyone you work with is just rooting for you. It was an extraordinary feeling of love I was surrounded with, and to this day, I'm very grateful for it.

I didn't know at the time that I only had four more weeks of pregnancy to go; I was still expecting to carry the boys until at least 37 weeks instead of the 34 weeks it turned out to be. For that last month before my babies were born, I was still working, but it was much less stressful. Every day someone helped me and my lounge chair (which I took everywhere, just in case) into the car and drove me to the studio, where I recorded the vocals for the *Dr. Quinn* shows. If you've never been on a movie set before, you might not know that the sound that's recorded while the actors are performing the scene is not always the sound you hear when the final movie is shown. The sound track needs to be cleaned up and actors re-record parts of it in a studio where there is much more control; so for example, the audience won't hear the airplane that happened to roar overhead during a *Dr. Quinn* scene!

Your Checkups

From the 30th week on, Dr. Ross continued to carefully check my weight gain. I was still struggling to eat more, and I was relieved when I stepped on the scales at her office one day to see that at last I'd gained a total of 38 pounds, just above the minimum of 35 pounds she'd prescribed for me.

More important even than adequate weight gain (which is *very* important), was her monitoring of my blood pressure and contractions. She explained that during the final weeks of a twin pregnancy it is vital to be especially watchful for hypertension of pregnancy, also known as preeclampsia.

By now, James and I were quite used to our routine of checking my contractions and my blood pressure for the final time each day before we went to bed. I'll admit that some nights it seemed like such a chore, it was the last thing I felt like doing. Sometimes I even dozed off before we did the blood pressure reading, and then James would wake me and I'd have to drag myself up to take it and send it in.

One night at 34 weeks was just like that. I don't remember what I'd done that day; but whatever it was, I was so thoroughly exhausted, it was about 11:00 P.M. and both James and I were tempted to skip the reading and do one first thing in the morning. In fact, one of us—probably me—said, "Oh, it's so late, let's just

What Are the Warning Signs of Preeclampsia?
Or Pregnancy-Induced Hypertension?

Preeclampsia, also known as toxemia, occurs in 10 to 25 percent of all pregnancies, but it is more common in twin pregnancies, first pregnancies and in women who have had high blood pressure, and it typically occurs during the second half of pregnancy. Its cause is unknown. A rapid rise in blood pressure and protein in the urine, usually along with one or more of the following symptoms characterize preeclampsia. Let your doctor know immediately if you experience any of these:

- Persistent headaches or dizziness.
- Visual disturbances or the sensation of flashing lights before your eyes.
- Rapid weight gain of more than a pound a day or three pounds in a week, along with puffiness of the hands, face or feet.
- Infrequent or inability to urinate.
- Stomach pains—not Braxton-Hicks contractions.
- Decrease in fetal movement.

forget about it and do it in the morning." But fortunately James and I tend to balance each other, and when one is feeling lazy, the other does the necessary prodding. We both knew we had to do the reading; to skip it would be irresponsible. So I did the reading myself after all, and the machine said my blood pressure was higher than usual. James took a look at it and said, "There must be something wrong with the machine—that number can't be right." So we waited a couple of minutes and tried again, but it was still a littler higher than it should have been. Now we were both nervous. A few minutes later we took my blood pressure once more, and it was the same.

I called Dr. Ross even though it was so late, and I told her about the blood pressure reading being higher than normal. She immediately asked if I had a headache or any visual changes, like seeing spots before my eyes, which she later explained are the classic questions a doctor asks to discern if blood pressure is really a problem. I hadn't had either of those symptoms, so we all felt relieved to know James and I could safely sleep that night at home. But we promised to see Dr. Ross at her office in the morning, first thing. After I hung up the phone, James and I fell into bed, thoroughly exhausted from all the uproar.

I was worried though. If my blood pressure didn't come down, I was certain that when we showed up for our checkup the next day that she was about to prescribe some form of bed rest. I

What Exactly Is Bed Rest?

So your doctor has told you that you're now to be on bed rest. Do you know exactly what that means? It pays to ask questions to be sure you and your doctor are on the same page. For example, do you know if it's all right to do light housework, such as vacuuming, at home? Can you drive yourself to the grocery store and shop? Can you sit up? How about walking up and down stairs? Taking a shower?

If you are going to be on bed rest for a few days, for weeks, or even for months, contact an organization called Sidelines (949–497–2265), a national support network for women with high-risk pregnancies, for detailed information on this and other issues.

fervently hoped if that was to be how I'd spend these last weeks of my pregnancy, she'd let me be on bed rest at home. I was at 34 weeks, and I didn't want to leave Katie and Sean until I was 36 to 38 weeks, which Dr. Ross considered term for twins. At the same time, I was so thankful that this was happening at 34 weeks, and not earlier. If the babies were born soon, which actually was the farthest thought from my mind (or maybe one I just didn't want to consider), it didn't seem terribly early. Maybe everything would turn out all right, I told myself as I drifted off to sleep that night.

All of these thoughts crowded through my weary brain as I tossed and turned, but not one of them completely prepared me for all that happened the next day.

Your Babies, As They Grow

As I gazed in wonder at my very large belly in the mirror each morning as I stepped out of the shower, I really loved to picture

What If My Babies Are Born in the Third Trimester?

Twins born after 29 weeks are slightly developmentally more mature, particularly in their lung development, than are third trimester singletons. It's not clear why this is true, and it should **not** be seen as a signal that it's fine for twins to be born any time during this trimester. Later is better!

Twins born between 29 and 32 weeks are considered early preterm for multiples. Most triplets and quadruplets are born during this time period, and often the outlook for them is good. Mothers of twins should shoot for several more weeks of pregnancy, even though by 32 weeks, the uterus of the our two boys curled inside. They were obviously so large (four or more pounds each, by Dr. Ross' estimate) that I couldn't feel as much dramatic movement as I had during the second trimester. Movement was an intense wriggling feeling now, still with significantly more activity on one side than on the other. Happily, ultrasounds had been showing for weeks that both boys were now head down, perfect for a vaginal birth.

Your Self, Your Family

This was a time when James and my children really became indispensable to me. I'm not used to leaning on people, but at this point I didn't have much choice, and I shall be eternally grateful for all they did. If there's one thing I saw with beautiful clarity during my twin pregnancy, it was how much my husband and children loved me and were willing to support me. As women, wives and mothers, many of us do shoulder a lot of responsibility

typical mother of twins is the same size as that of a singleton mom at full term.

Twins born between 33 and 35 weeks are considered preterm for multiples. As many as half of twins are born during this time period. Most of these twins spend a week or two in the hospital and go home without lasting ill effects.

Your ultimate goal should be to get to 36–38 weeks, which is the time period considered to be term for twins. Born at term, your babies are more likely to be comparable in health to a singleton, and they're likely to be able to go home from the hospital with you. The average birth weight for twins is five and a half pounds each.

at home and in our careers. While I found it difficult to let go of some of that sense of responsibility, even late in my pregnancy, the end result was that it was a tremendous opportunity to learn about myself, and to let those around me share the load. It was a gift, actually, for all of us.

How Will I Survive Prolonged Bed Rest?

It's a big help if you can learn to rely on others for more support than you may be used to. Here are a few suggestions to get you started:

- Make a list of things people can do for you, so when they ask, you have something to tell them.
- Get household and child care help. If you can't afford it, ask coworkers, friends, church members, to help you out with these things.
- Ask friends to bring meals.
- Invite someone to visit, when you feel up to it.
- Scan the phone book for grocery stores, pharmacies and restaurants that deliver.

We all worry about how to make sure our other children will still feel important when twins arrive. And because I simply couldn't carry on as if nothing were happening, I stumbled on one of the simplest and most effective ways to include my other children. I asked them to help me! Sometimes it was just to be with me, to keep me company as I rested. Sometimes I needed an extra pair of hands to lift the lounge chair, lightweight though it was, into the car. Before my eyes I could see that each of my children felt the importance of what they did for me, and I knew that simply by needing them, I was helping them reaffirm their value and their place in our family.

The Straight Scoop:
Notes for Dads from James

Jane's irritable uterus and the terbutaline pump she came home with marked a turning point for me in her pregnancy. While I had been closely involved from the beginning, going to all the doctor's visits with her and all the sonogram visits, I knew that this complication was my cue to check in with the doctor on my own. It was one of the things I could do to keep track of what was happening, to help the doctor manage the pregnancy, and to keep a little bit of the responsibility off Jane's shoulders.

So for all that time Jane was on the terbutaline pump, I'd call the doctor every day to be sure I had a clear view of the big picture. I came to think of it as similar to someone calling a stockbroker every day to see how he's doing—and checking on the numbers. "Where are we with the numbers?" I'd ask Dr. Ross, and she'd let me know about Jane's blood pressure and the contractions and any trends she saw in either of those.

I kept myself prepared to go to the hospital at any time. Jane didn't know this then, but I had a little emergency bag packed and in the car weeks earlier than we'd need it. It's just my nature to be prepared, but I think it's good advice to dads. You can be on top of the situation if you're always one step ahead, and at some point, your wife may need you to be one step ahead.

Not only was I prepared, but I was optimistic. Maybe that's just my nature too, but I always felt that in spite of the crises we faced, everything was going to turn out all right. As her pregnancy wore on, I think Jane came to rely more and more on me for my good attitude. Not that she lacked strength! Jane, she's mighty. I used to call her the Mighty Quinn! But when she was pregnant, I wanted to take away the whirlwind of activity that is the usual state of our household. I wanted to protect her from worries as much as possible, to keep things calm for her so she could put her focus where it really belonged—on growing the babies.

I'd also write her love letters and send them by fax. We did that before we were married—we had a courtship by fax. Late in her pregnancy I started writing little notes again, thanking her for doing this for me and for the babies, telling her how much I loved her, how beautiful she was to me. Writing this down, I realized more fully how much this pregnancy and these babies were a gift from her to me. I began to see it all personally, as a personal gift to me. And to see that there could be no greater gift for us to share, than our children.

Writing Jane these romantic notes, making sure the house was always filled with flowers Jane loved, checking in with the doctor—these things were the least I could do in return for the physical and emotional stress Jane went through during this pregnancy.

While I never had to be on full bed rest, I have friends who were. I know there are days we all have when we wish someone would tell us to go to our room and rest, just like we'd tell a grumpy five-year-old to do. But after seeing my friend endure weeks of being confined to her room, and hearing about the aches and pains that inactivity can bring and the side effects of the medication she was taking to keep labor away, I knew that bed rest can be far from relaxing. She did end up with two beautiful, healthy little girls born at 35 weeks, so it was worth every minute of difficulty the bed rest presented. But I could see how hard it was for her. If you've been assigned to bed rest, my advice is to get in touch with an organization called Sidelines (949–497–2265). It's a national support network for women who are in the midst of high-risk pregnancies. They helped my friend with advice and put her in contact with another woman who'd been through the same thing, and I know they can help you.

Looking Good, Feeling Good

Even though you've probably adjusted your attitude about what constitutes looking good, it becomes more of a challenge in the last weeks of your pregnancy. Everything about your body is probably becoming just too much. Too much belly, too much bosom, to say the least. I have friends who actually grew out of all their maternity clothing before the end of their twin pregnancy.

My advice is to be prepared. In these last weeks, most of us aren't exactly social butterflies, so your wardrobe needs have probably shrunk with your activity level. Still, I'd suggest you take a look in your closet and check out the clothing you wear most often. Try on the basics you depend upon, and estimate which are likely to go the distance with you. I felt so much better being certain I had a few things I knew would fit me and look decent, rather than risking an unpleasant surprise as I tried to squeeze into something that no longer fit, minutes before I was supposed to walk out the door.

I also started relying more often on my favorite pregnancy accessories: large scarves and shawls. They are a great way to add some glamour or softness to an outfit, and you can use lovely colors that compliment your own coloring. Best of all, they do soften the silhouette and draw the eye upward.

Dressing Well

One thing that took me a little by surprise very late in my pregnancy, was a request from *TV Guide* magazine to do a cover shoot of me in all my glory. I wasn't working any more by that time, so it seemed like a reasonably enjoyable outing during which I would only have to stand up for a few minutes at a time. My only hesitation was that I didn't think they'd have clothing that would fit me and that would be flattering. So once again I called on Cheri, and told her my worries about the shoot. Somehow, the day before the shoot, she managed to get into the studio where we would be to take a look at the clothing the stylist was providing. What she found was exactly what we were afraid of. The stylist, while a very talented woman, had never had kids and the clothing she brought reflected the fact that she didn't understand the sensitivities that a pregnant woman would have, nor the size she would need!

Cheri reported that the clothing was what a fashion model, pregnant with one baby, might have chosen: short dresses revealing the belly, a little low cut and showing a lot of bosom. While both Cheri and I agree there is a lot of sensuality in pregnancy, fortunately we also agreed that the crucial question is, how much do you show and still look attractive rather than sloppy?

After her visit to the studio, without my even knowing it, Cheri went out and found some fabric to make something for me, overnight!

The next day, she walked into the shoot and casually asked me, "So, how are you doing?"

"Oh," I grumbled, "they're still trying to find something that fits me."

"How about this?" she asked, and held up the most gorgeous burgundy gown. It was made of a luscious stretch velour. She'd given the dress a medieval look with a lovely drape in the front, a train in the back, long sleeves coming down on the hand and a bit of drape at the top of the arm. The instant I put it on, I felt beautiful and regal, and we found some fabulous jewelry to wear with it. Talk about a friend being a true lifesaver!

In creating that dress, Cheri had used all the principles for looking good we'd discussed earlier in my pregnancy. The stretchy fabric had enough weight and give so that it would fall beautifully, and even though I was only weeks away from giving birth, it made me look graceful rather than just huge. All during my pregnancy my growth had been mostly out in front, but now I was getting bigger around the sides too, but the drape of the dress accommodated that. A little extra room in the upper arms disguised how spindly my arms had become as my belly had grown, but it could just as well have disguised upper arms that have become heavier, which is what happens to many women. And the color was rich and flattering, with enough detail at the neckline to draw the eye upward. The end result: one of my favorite magazine cover shots on the November 25–December 1, 1996 cover of *TV Guide*.

The one social event I really wanted to dress for late in my pregnancy was the baby shower we had at home. Again, it was Cheri and her advice to the rescue. I wore a simple short black dress similar to something I'd wear if I weren't pregnant, with black hose and shoes to keep from chopping my body into awkward color blocks. Over the dress I wore a colorful silk Chinese jacket, again, something I'd wear pregnant or not. I loved the softness of the silk jacket. Of course nothing hides your belly at this point, but like a shawl or scarf, the silk jacket provided an illusion of lightness. I felt truly lovely that evening. Of course that evening I was parked in my chaise lounge, and wasn't allowed to move at all. All my doctors were there, hovering over me. I knew they'd become very nervous if I got up to greet guests and shake hands with everyone, so I just stayed put. One of my best friends is Christopher Reeve, ever since we made the movie "Somewhere In Time" together years ago. As I sat there, strange as it may sound, I thought of Chris, and that this is a little of what he must feel like now, being in a wheelchair and having no control over where you go.

This wasn't a surprise shower, and this one wasn't so much about the gifts and gathering of needed equipment. James and some of my friends planned it as a special celebration of the impending birth of our twins, but I had no idea it would be such a spectacular evening. A real high point was the cake—or rather the two cakes—Candace and Steve Garvey supplied. They were in the shape of two toddlers wearing baseball outfits, complete with a pair of real autographed baseballs and bats from Steve.

As you can see from my experience, how you plan a baby shower, who plans it, why you have one, and even *whether* you'll have one are all questions to which you can find your own answers. I know some people feel it's bad luck to gear up for the babies before they're born. If that's the case for your family, it's easy enough to send your husband out to pick up some diapers and undershirts for them after they're born, while you're still all in the hospital.

Exercise

With modifications provided by my trainer Birgitta Gallo and Dr. Ross, I exercised right up to the day my boys were born. Notice I said with *modifications!* Any exercise program, particularly a program undertaken when you are pregnant with twins, must be given the go-ahead, and then monitored, by your doctor. Even if you have been exercising right along, by this time in your pregnancy it's a good idea to once again check in with your doctor. You may want to change your routine now to accommodate your increasing size, or your doctor may want you to stop exercising altogether to avoid preterm labor or other complications. I have one friend who found that certain movements that didn't bother her earlier in the pregnancy seemed to stimulate contractions once she got bigger. We laughed because one of those movements was the pulling and pushing that comes with vacuuming. Too bad. She had a hard time explaining to her husband that while she could still lift certain weights in her workout, she couldn't vacuum the living room floor!

My workout stayed essentially the same between 28 and 34 weeks, with some important exceptions because of the irritable uterus episode I'd had at 28 weeks. I no longer warmed up on either the recumbent bike or the StairMaster. I also used stretchy exercise bands instead of the weight machine, and I did exercises seated or lying down instead of standing. Gently, I kept up with my abdominal exercises, even though I had grown so large, although Dr. Ross pointed out that if I had experienced pre-term labor, all abdominal exercises would have been out. At this point I started doing simple isometrics, pulling my abdominal muscles inward and holding them for a count of 10. Even that was difficult, but I really felt that keeping those muscles, which were under so much stress, as toned as possible would help me feel better while I was pregnant and help me to recover faster afterward. I did do a few abdominal curls, and Birgitta showed me how to cross my arms over my belly, or to simply place a hand on either side of my belly to support those muscles by gently pushing them toward an imaginary line running down the center of my belly. She cautioned me that straining without support could result in pulling apart the two large vertical sheets of muscle that make up the abdominals, which can weaken them after the pregnancy. So I was careful about supporting those muscles.

I also knew it was important to keep up with my upper back and shoulder exercises for the same reason. Those muscles were under stress too, and the stronger they were, the less my back hurt.

After I had that irritable uterus episode at 28 weeks, I also reviewed with Birgitta what I would do if Dr. Ross said I had to go on bed rest. I was relieved to know that many of the exercises I had been doing could be done in another way even if I was confined to bed, using the stretchy exercise bands for my arms and back, and staying away from abdominal exercises of any kind. Of course if I had been on bed rest, I would have checked with Dr. Ross before I did anything, but it was good to know that I would have some options.

Can I Exercise If I'm on Bed Rest?

Depending on what your doctor says, there are exercises that can be done even if you are on bed rest. In fact, you may have fewer of the aches and pains that can come with inactivity if you do a few (doctor approved) bed rest exercises.

Work with your doctor and a personal trainer experienced in helping pregnant women to develop a program that's right for you. Here are some ideas:

- You can always do Kegels.
- If you do have an **approved** exercise routine, do seated exercises first, focusing on shoulders and back, then do all the side-lying exercises (for legs and hips) on one side before you do all the side-lying exercises on the other side. Turning over is exercise in itself, so you'll want to minimize the number of times you do that. If you're not allowed to sit up, do the exercises and stretches you can lying on your side or briefly on your back, if your doctor approves.
- If you are strong enough and your doctor approves, add exercise bands, light dumbbells or light ankle weights to your routine.
- Don't do any exercise or movement that makes your uterus contract!

BED REST EXERCISE ROUTINE

Upper Body

Lat pull: Sitting up straight in bed, hold a stretchy exercise band by the handles so it is in front of you. Pull your arms apart and back, squeezing your shoulder blades together. Slowly return to starting position. Repeat 10 to 20 times.

Rowing: Sitting up straight in bed, loop an exercise band around your feet. Pull both elbows back, squeezing your shoulder blades together. Slowly return to beginning position. Repeat 10 to 20 times. This can also be done lying on your side, one elbow at a time, with no exercise band.

Chest press: Sitting up straight in bed, loop exercise band around your back and hold the ends at your chest. Press your hands forward, flexing your chest muscles. Release slowly. Repeat 10 to 20 times.

Lower Body

Leg extension: Sit up straight in bed with knees bent and pillows under knees. Keeping knees together, extend the right leg out straight, flex the thigh muscles and hold for a second. Release. Repeat 10 to 20 times on each leg.

Leg lifts: Lie on your right side with the right leg bent for support, left leg straight with the foot flexed. Bend the left leg to flex the hamstring, lifting it slightly and moving the knee back a few inches by flexing the buttock. Hold for a few seconds, then release. Repeat on each side 10 to 20 times.

Lie in the same position, but slowly raise the left leg up about 12 inches, and slowly lower it. Repeat 10 to 20 times on each side. Use a light ankle weight if you are strong enough.

Hip opener: Lie on your right side, both knees bent to a 90-degree angle in front of you. Lift your left knee until it is perpendicular to the bed, opening the hip joint. Slowly release. Repeat 10 to 20 times on each side.

Abdominal Exercises

Crunch: Sit up in bed or lie on your side. Placing your hands on your belly as in the illustration on page 73, contract the muscles as tight as you can, rounding your back. Release and straighten your back. Repeat 10 to 20 times.

Stretches

Gentle stretches you are familiar with can be done in bed. Here are a few to try:

Elbow chest stretch: Sitting in bed, place both hands behind your head. Gently press your elbows backward, stretching shoulders and chest muscles.

Triceps stretch: Sit up straight in bed, and lift your right arm up behind your head. Holding your right elbow with your left hand, stretch your right hand down your back until you feel a gentle stretch in your triceps. Repeat on the other side.

Hamstring stretch: Sit up or lie on your right side with your right knee bent for support. Hold your left ankle or calf with your left hand, keeping the leg as straight as possible. Repeat on the other side.

Details

If you're not one of those lucky women who have that glowing skin during their pregnancy, you have plenty of company. Some women seem to get a blotchy look, with tiny broken blood vessels you can see on the surface. Most likely those are from the increased blood supply we all have during pregnancy, and for the most part they disappear after the babies are born. I would think a good cover-up would take care of some of the blotches until then.

Another unwelcome skin change that some women experience is one that my mother called "the mask of pregnancy." It consists of brownish dark spots that can appear on the face during pregnancy. I didn't get these, but I asked Dr. Ross about them since I knew that with twins I was likely to have more of everything, and perhaps that would include those spots. She explained the spots were just another result of pregnancy hormones at work, and that if I got them, they would go away after the birth. Even though I'd never had them in my previous pregnancies, I planned ahead in a couple of ways, just in case. I was prepared to cover any splotches with makeup, and I increased the SPF of the sunscreen I normally use, because Dr. Ross told me that sun exposure may make them worse.

The other skin change I did get was that dark brown line down the center of my belly. I think it appeared at around five months or so, but it was quite distinct. It's also the result of all those pregnancy hormones. To be honest, I didn't do anything special about it—in fact there's nothing you can do about it. I just moisturized like I always do, and just as Dr. Ross said it would, it disappeared within weeks of the babies' birth.

You're almost there! I hope you're taking life very easy now, watching and waiting, and staying in close contact with your doctor. Set aside a quiet evening at home alone with your husband. It's a great time to tell him how much you appreciate him.

Checklist for Late Pregnancy

Begin:

- Collecting clothing and equipment you'll need. (See Chapter 7 for ideas.)
- Reviewing your plans for the birth. Talk with your doctor about whether you're likely to have a cesarean section or a vaginal birth, and how you feel about each.
- Making a list of people you will want to contact with news when the babies are born.
- Making arrangements for child care for your other children for when the babies are born.
- Thinking about whether you'll want or need help when you come home with two newborns, and make arrangements for it. (See Chapter 6 for ideas.)

Phase out:

- Working! Arrange for your leave of absence if you plan to return to work later.
- Running around in general. Allow your babies to have the benefit of these last weeks in the womb, and allow yourself to have the rest you need.
- Worrying about your pregnancy. You're almost finished!

five

Giving Birth

For months—although it may seem longer—you've been looking ahead to the day when your babies would, at last, be born. And here you are; your babies' birthday is very close indeed. I, like you, was *so* excited and impatient to finally meet those little ones. No matter how excited you are though, when you think about their birth, you may find there's also a scary little voice in the back of your head that keeps repeating phrases like, "What if . . . ?" and "How will I . . . ?"

I've heard that unsettling voice, too. Although I'd given birth twice before and was an experienced mom, those other births were not twin births. Those babies came to me one at a time, and even so, I knew that during each of their births or right afterwards, there had been moments when it all seemed so overwhelming. I couldn't help but think, *What is going to happen when I give birth to twins?* While I certainly knew I'd be having these twins one at a time, still I felt a bit in the dark about the details of exactly how the birth would happen and how I would care for both of them afterwards. There were some very fundamental questions whirling around in my head, starting with, "Am I having a cesarean or am I having a vaginal birth?"

In order to feel at peace with it all, I found that I needed to know everything I could about what was likely to happen during this birth, no matter what type it would be. For me, and perhaps for you, too, knowledge is the key. For example, before one knows anything about it, it's easy to think, "Oh no, a cesarean! That's pretty radical!" But I'd had the privilege when I was a girl in England, about 10 years old, of going to an operating theatre with my father to actually watch a cesarean being performed. My father was an obstetrician, and through watching various surgeries with him, I developed a keen appreciation for how brilliantly the human body is designed. Of course that experience is not available to everyone, nor is everyone likely to be interested in watching surgery. But I think because I knew exactly what happened during a cesarean, it wasn't so strange to me when we discussed the possibility with Dr. Ross months before the babies' birth. You can put yourself in that position by talking in detail with your doctor and by reading up on cesareans in medically oriented pregnancy books your doctor recommends.

I will admit though, that it's possible one can have too much knowledge. On the day I was 34 weeks pregnant and Dr. Ross had me admitted to the hospital because of my high blood pressure, that was the day I first realized it would most likely be *me* having a cesarean this time, and I was genuinely frightened at first. But eventually, given a little time to get used to the idea, knowing about cesareans did help make the possibility that I would have one a little less scary.

For my earlier births, there was no question that I'd have a vaginal birth each time. With Katie, who was born in 1982, my husband and I were eager to attend Lamaze classes, hungry for every detail. I thought about having an underwater birth, or at least a birth that would take place somewhere calm and beautiful, like in a lovely room with lace curtains. At that time everyone wanted to give birth anywhere except in a hospital. My father the obstetrician however, was quite adamant about a hospital being the best place for me to have my baby, and he was coming from England to be with me for the birth. So I compromised by bring-

Cesarean Birth or Vaginal Birth?

About half of twin pregnancies end in cesarean births and the other half are vaginal. If you are having triplets or more, you can be pretty sure you're going to have them by cesarean. But if you're having twins, it's not so clear which type of birth it will be. Often, even the doctor doesn't know which it will be until you are in labor.

Having babies, even twins, the old-fashioned way, vaginally, generally means you'll have a lower risk of infection, less bleeding and a quicker recovery. Whether a vaginal birth is right for you and your babies depends on your medical status at the time, on your medical history (for example whether you've had a cesarean or a vaginal birth previously) and on the babies' position when you go into labor.

If they're both head down and you've had a healthy, uneventful pregnancy, you're likely to at least have a trial of labor to see if it progresses well enough to have a vaginal birth. If the baby nearest the cervix is head down and the second baby is not, you may still be able to have a vaginal birth. The cervix usually remains fully dilated, or nearly so, for some time after the birth of the first baby, which may allow the doctor to adjust the position of the second baby if it is transverse (crossways) or breech (feet or bottom first). Occasionally, the first twin is born vaginally and because of the position of the second baby or another complication, the second one needs to be born by cesarean.

If you've had a cesarean birth before, you'll need to talk to your doctor about whether you can have a vaginal birth with twins.

ing as many lovely, soft things as I could with me to the hospital to make it seem less like an institution and more like home.

As it turned out though, I was very glad I was in a good hospital when Katie was born. On her way out, she pushed her fist right through my rectal wall, which required an enormous amount of fancy stitch work to repair. I was grateful to my father for convincing me to have Katie in a place where difficulties like this could be easily handled. And I was grateful to the doctor who didn't make a huge fuss about it when it happened. I'd had an epidural, so I didn't feel it, but the doctor was also careful not to interfere with me having that most amazing moment on earth, of knowing I'd given birth to my daughter.

I think that experience, in which I'd had to be open to options other than what I had planned for, prepared me well for my twins' birth. By the end of my twin pregnancy, I was truly ready for whatever kind of birth would be right for the babies. If it would be better for them that I have a cesarean rather than a vaginal birth, which I would have preferred, then so be it. Besides, everything else about the conception and the pregnancy so far had involved choices I never dreamed I'd be making, so I began to assume the birth, too, would probably involve choices I hadn't planned on.

In order to feel truly confident about whatever was going to happen during the birth, I found I also needed to talk to someone about exactly how either type would likely go. Dr. Ross was a great help in that regard, and of course James was as well. I'm sure James must have gotten sick of hearing me go on, but he never complained when I wanted to discuss, over and over, the steps in a twin birth. He must have realized that it was somehow calming to me. As a result, I found that the more I talked about the coming birth, the more whatever remaining fears or concerns I had bubbled to the surface, and the more likely I was to feel comforted and to get answers to my what-if and how-will-I questions. Finally, by the time I was about 32 weeks pregnant, I arrived at that point where the idea of physically giving birth to two babies no longer seemed strange and fearsome to me. It seemed downright do-able!

We also had a childbirth educator come to our house for a one evening refresher course at about that time. I was supposed to be on at least partial bed rest, so we were lucky to find someone who would accommodate us at home. No matter whether you're expecting a cesarean or a vaginal birth, I highly recommend taking a class if you haven't, or attending a refresher if you have. And, if there is a special childbirth preparation class in your area for those expecting a multiple birth, sign up for it! Whether or not you are an experienced parent, classes like these can give you and your partner something to think about, new questions to ask your doctor—and in the end, an extra measure of confidence. You'll also meet other expectant parents, which is great. You're not alone, you know! Even though James and I felt that we already knew some of what the childbirth educator talked about, having her here did make us really tune in, to think ahead to the reality of meeting these babies. It opened the door for us to this last phase of pregnancy, and we really began preparing in our hearts and minds for the birth.

In the end, it was James who provided me with the foundation for a calm perspective. He reminded me that the babies' birth would be just a few hours out of their (and our) whole lives, and that we had a great team of doctors to take care of me, and the babies during those hours. Most importantly, he reassured me repeatedly that we *had* done all we could to give the babies a healthy start in life. I still worried at times that I hadn't done quite enough; that I'd worked too long, too hard, and too far into my pregnancy. But James also reminded me that now, when we were so close to the boys' birth, it was time to move beyond whatever regret I might have about what I did or didn't do during my pregnancy. "Stay 'in the present moment' with the babies," he said, "and do the best you can right now, *today*."

He was so right, but I'm sure neither of us had any idea how much his words were to help me through what quickly became the last, and harrowing, days of my pregnancy.

Your Pregnant Body

As James and I drove to Dr. Ross' office on November 29, 1995, the day I was 34 weeks pregnant, I had a sinking feeling that I wasn't going to make it to my gestation goal. I'd wanted the babies to have 37 weeks inside before they were born. After hearing the serious tone in Dr. Ross' voice the night before when we'd discussed my slightly elevated blood pressure, I could picture that goal going up in smoke.

It wasn't so much that I was worried about myself during our drive to her office; my mind was on the babies. If my blood pressure wouldn't settle down, were they ready to be born? Would they pay a price for my competitive nature, for my sense of responsibility to my work on the show and to the crew? I can only describe my feelings as the beginnings of remorse. I said a silent prayer that they wouldn't be coming out too soon, and if they had to, that they would be healthy.

Dr. Ross ushered us immediately into her office. After she checked my blood pressure, she stood back and looked at me for a moment. "I hate to say it," she said, "but I've been waiting for this to happen, because it's so common in women of your age who are having twins." She paused before adding, "You have mild preeclampsia."

As James and I listened, she went on to explain that my very pregnant body was sending signals—loud and clear—that it had had enough. My blood pressure had continued to rise, and a urine test showed there was protein in my urine. Both were signs of mild preeclampsia, a condition potentially dangerous both to myself and to the babies. Dr. Ross told me she would be admitting me to the hospital immediately. She wanted to see if she could get my blood pressure to come down, to conduct tests that would show if the babies could safely be born now, and to have blood work done on me to check on the function of my organs. Left untreated, preeclampsia would eventually affect the function of my liver and kidneys, she said.

The only bright note was that Dr. Ross reassured us that the cure for preeclampsia was delivery of the babies. It wasn't a long discussion, but it was a terrifying one. Before we could completely digest what she'd said, I was whisked off to a room in Santa Monica hospital, which is near her office building.

I think I kept myself calm that day by focusing on the mundane, thinking about little things like the hospital bag and what was in it. I knew James had already packed one for me, and that he'd stowed it in the car weeks ago in case we'd had a premature birth. I was glad for his foresight, and fussing over that detail put the immediate fear out of my mind for a few minutes. Normally, I didn't care much about what would be in that bag. After having a couple of babies, I've come to think that too much is made about what to take to the hospital. After all, when you're giving birth, you're in a hospital gown for the longest time, and if you're anything like me, you don't really care! In most cases, you can send someone to the hospital gift shop or home to retrieve anything that's been forgotten. The one exception is warm socks. With each birth I did make sure I had a pair of big woolly socks to wear while I was having the baby. My feet easily get really cold, so the socks definitely contributed to my comfort.

Other than socks, in my opinion there are only two other essential pieces of equipment: one is that you must have plenty of cameras (video and still) to record the great moments, and the other is that you must have music that you love. I'd wanted a particular piece of music that was very special to me: the music from the romantic movie I made years ago with Christopher Reeve, "Somewhere In Time," which was composed by John Barry, a friend of ours.

By two that afternoon, I had settled into the plain little hospital room, gladly climbing into bed to rest. Within a couple of hours, Dr. Connie Agnew, the neonatologist we'd seen early in the pregnancy, came to do an amniocentesis to check on the maturity of the boys' lungs, which would tell us if the boys would be all right if they were in fact born that day. Thankfully, the test showed the boys were about four pounds each, big enough to be born, and that their lungs were mature. I can assure you, that news was a huge relief to me and to James.

But unfortunately, that piece of good news didn't have anything to do with my blood pressure. Instead of dropping into the normal range as we'd hoped it would, it continued to climb. By 11:00 that night, blood tests showed that my liver function had begun to deteriorate. Of course I wasn't particularly aware of either of those details at the time. I found out days later that through the night, Dr. Ross and James had several corridor conferences and whispered conversations, none of which included me. They went to great lengths to keep me from being aware of the seriousness of the drama being played out in my body as the preeclampsia progressed from the mild form to the severe form. Later Dr. Ross explained that when she saw that my liver function tests were abnormal, although they weren't great, she felt there was still time for me to have the babies vaginally. Near midnight, she started me on an IV with pitocin, a synthetic form of the hormone oxytocin, which causes labor contractions, in order to see if my labor would begin. At the same time, she also started magnesium sulfate, which can help lower blood pressure, but more importantly also is an antiseizure drug. One of the dangers of severe preeclampsia is that the mother can have seizures or even a stroke.

I'm so glad I didn't know any of this at the time. This was one case when for me, more knowledge would definitely have *not* been better. I don't generally like people to keep things from me, but as I got sicker, that's exactly what they did. They simply took care of me as they would a child—with kindness and tenderness, but without explaining the scary parts in too much detail. After the boys were born and I heard what had actually happened that night, I was grateful that Dr. Ross and James had kept the facts about my failing health from me at the moment, and that by doing so, neither of them produced an atmosphere of crisis around me. I don't think I could have handled it—my blood pressure was high enough! James and Dr. Ross really created a kind of quiet cocoon for me.

It made sense to me that Dr. Ross would induce my labor and try for a vaginal birth, because I'd had two babies already, and we both knew that the recovery from a vaginal birth is generally easier than recovery from a cesarean. Besides, she also knew that being induced was quite familiar to me. I have never had a baby—

singleton or twin—who wanted to come out. I am the queen of inductions! Katie, my oldest, was two and a half weeks late. I don't know if it was that she simply had her own time schedule or that she was just so comfortable that she didn't want to leave the womb, but we did end up inducing her. After the long wait for Katie, I asked to be induced on my due date with Sean. Now here I was again, in different circumstances indeed, but still being induced. "Some things never change," I thought as I tried to make myself comfortable with the pitocin IV in my arm.

What Causes Labor to Begin, and How Will I Know It Has Started?

We know the symptoms of labor, but strangely enough, we don't completely understand what triggers the symptoms. Here are things to look for to tell you if labor is about to start:

- **Bloody show:** This happens when the mucous plug that has sealed the entrance to the uterus comes out because the cervix has begun to open and thin out. The plug is made of a slightly bloody gel-like material.
- **Rupture of membranes:** This is when the amniotic sac in which your babies have been floating, either breaks with a splash of fluid on the floor, or springs a leak that dribbles fluid out slowly.
- **Uterine contractions:** These are stronger and more regular than the Braxton-Hicks, or practice contractions you may have been feeling for a while. A rule of thumb is that if the contractions are regular, if they continue even when you try to rest, and if you feel them in your back as well as your abdomen, you may be in labor and you should check with your doctor.

The next morning, November 30, Dr. Ross checked on me to see how my labor was progressing, and I was a little discouraged to hear that almost nothing had changed—I was a mere 2 centimeters dilated. Dr. Ross broke one of the two bags of waters, which often brings on contractions. Fortunately, the magnesium sulfate had helped my blood pressure to level off, so she decided to wait a while longer to see if my labor would pick up. At 3:00 in the afternoon, after a long, tedious day, still nothing was happening. Although I wasn't fearful—that calm, focused feeling prevailed—at the same time, I wasn't surprised when Dr. Ross sat on my bed, took my hand, smiled down at me and said, "I think we're going to do a cesarean."

I smiled back and said, "Oh really? When?"

"Now," she answered sweetly.

"Okay. Now," I responded. It was all so simple.

Later she explained to me that the only real change that had occurred overnight was that I was getting sicker at a faster rate. The babies needed to come into the world as soon as possible, in order to take the stress off my body.

James' mother and father had come to the hospital to see us that morning, and of course Katie and Sean had been with me all day, keeping me company. Sean would tell silly jokes to make me laugh; Katie would refill my water jug or just sit holding my hand. Once the cesarean decision had been made though, in an instant it seemed the anesthesiologist was in my room, explaining what he was about to do. Although I am a great fan of epidurals, I'm not a fan of the moment they are administered. Of course we had everyone except James leave the room. It was quite difficult for me with my huge belly to bend forward the way you have to, but not impossible. James was sitting next to me on the bed, stroking me gently on my face, my arms. There's something so soothing about the touch of a loved one. Touch is a powerful force—you feel that energy and that calming and healing from the other person, and somehow you're not so alone with whatever it is you have to deal with.

I have no doubt that James' touch helped me deal with the needle they use to administer the epidural. I have a theory about needles—if I don't see them, I'm okay. Just don't show me that needle! I also use a little diversion tactic: I jam my fingernail into my palm and concentrate on that—on the pain I *can* control. It helps me deal with the pain I can't control. Happily the pain of getting the epidural is over in a very few minutes; and truly, the idea of it is worse than any pain it causes. Then the kids were back in the room and before I knew it, it was hugs and kisses all around and I was off.

If you have a cesarean with your twins, your birth may be something like mine. Then again, it may be completely different. If there's one thing I've learned after having four children, it's that each birth is its own event, and like snowflakes, no two are exactly alike. Still, I think that there are similarities of procedure and of the feelings surrounding birth. If it can help you anticipate, or even make sense of your own cesarean birth of twins, I'm happy to share the details of my birth with you.

When Dr. Ross was ready for me, my whole bed was wheeled right into the operating room where I was transferred to an operating table and draped with what felt like an entire linen closet worth of sheets. It's so strange to look back at those photographs and the video James shot. They all show me smiling blissfully, as if I were doing nothing more dramatic than lying in bed. And indeed, I remember feeling quite happy and content. They must have given me a bit of a sedative, but I didn't feel drowsy or drugged. I think there were other reasons for my calm. Perhaps it was because I knew so much about cesareans and I was truly at peace with the idea of having one myself. Or maybe it was because I had been through so many medical procedures already, it didn't feel all that strange to be undergoing yet another one, and I just accepted it. I am also the eternal optimist, and I simply had to believe I was about to experience the happy ending to this pregnancy.

As I lay in the operating room waiting for Dr. Ross to begin, I listened to the voices of what sounded like dozens of people preparing for this birth. Because of the drape in front of my face that kept me from watching my own cesarean, I couldn't see anyone unless he or she stood right over my face, which no one except the anesthesiologist was doing. Still, I could tell from the sound that there were a lot of people in the room, and I remember thinking there wasn't going to be any intimate birth moment today. That is typical though, with a multiple birth. For each baby, there's usually a pediatrician or neonatologist along with one or two pediatric nurses. In our case, Dr. Lisa Stern, our pediatrician, was there to take care of both babies. Then there's the obstetrician and a second doctor assisting, along with a couple of surgical nurses. Dr. Paulson, the fertility specialist we worked with in order to get pregnant in the first place was there, too. I was glad to see him, but surprised as well—the fertility specialist usually doesn't show up at births. I suppose he'd seen us in his office so often, crying our eyes out after each miscarriage, that he wanted to see the happy outcome. At one point I could hear several people laughing and noting that he and James were the only men in the room, and idle observers at that. The nurses kept laughingly shooing them away, saying "Go over there now, stay out of the way so we women can get on with the work!"

But James stayed by my side the whole time, sitting at my head. If he hadn't been, I think the drape that blocked my vision would have made me feel a little isolated. I couldn't tell what was happening with the surgery at all. I have a girlfriend who told me she had two people with her during her cesarean: a friend and her husband. One of them could tell her what was happening and the other could take pictures, which seemed like a good idea. However James handled both for me. He kept one hand on my face, stroking my forehead or my cheek, and the other on a video camera, as he taped everything. Of course he's a movie director, so he *had* to have control of the camera! I could feel some pulling and tugging during the surgery, certainly no pain, but I had no idea what any of it meant. I kept asking James, "Have we got babies yet? Have we got babies?" He'd answer, "In a minute, they're washing your abdomen first," or "No babies yet sweetie, she's just starting the incision." I was surprised at how long it took to make the incision. Later Dr. Ross reminded me the incisions she made went through a single layer at a time, whether it was tissue or muscle or the uterus, so it's not just one big swipe with a scalpel. As she was working on me, at one point she exclaimed, "Great tissue Jane; a surgeon's dream," and later she said, "Look at those abdominal muscles—good work Jane. They look like the muscles of a 20-year old!" I can't take credit for whatever kind of tissue I have that makes it a surgeon's dream, but I'll admit to a certain amount of pride when she complimented me on my abs!

James filmed everything. He'd point the camera over the drape, keep it on what Dr. Ross was doing until he'd start to feel queasy, then he'd sweep the camera back to my face. The music from "Somewhere In Time" was playing in the background. I lay there telling myself, "This is it, the dramatic ending to this pregnancy. This is *it*." But somehow as I listened to the cordial banter and laughter floating in and out of the music, I had this surreal sense that it was really just a casual afternoon gathering of friends. What an odd feeling it was to sense that everything was at the same moment, perfectly ordinary, and absolutely extraordinary.

Once the incision had gone through the uterus, I could hear the liquid sounds of Dr. Ross suctioning out the amniotic fluid. At last it was time for the first baby to emerge! In our case, that was Johnny. After all those months of waiting, suddenly, there he was! Dr. Ross lifted him out and held him up like a trophy for me to admire. In a quick glimpse I could see Johnny's arms and legs waving furiously, his little face red and contorted as he screamed heartily. I thought he was perfectly adorable. A nurse whisked him away and about a minute later, there was Kris, not screaming but sort of mewling like a kitten. James and I were beside ourselves with joy. I could hear the tears in his voice as he kept saying, "They're so beautiful honey, so beautiful." Then he was kissing me, and we were both telling the boys, whom I couldn't see any more because of the drape, "Happy birthday!" and "Welcome." They were born at 4:02 and 4:03 in the afternoon.

As soon as they could, the nurses wrapped both boys warmly in receiving blankets and darling little knit hats, and held them where I could give them each a welcome-to-the-world kiss. Afterward the nurses took them both to the neonatal intensive care unit where they could be closely observed. Then it seemed to take forever to deliver the placentas and close the incision. I was so calm, so mellow, I didn't really mind, although I was eager to see my babies again, and I really wanted to see Katie and Sean. Luckily, just when I was beginning to feel a bit impatient, Dr. Ross said she was finished. All told, the surgery took about an hour, with the babies being born within about the first 15 minutes.

How Is a Vaginal Birth of Twins Different from a Singleton's Birth?

A lot of what happens in a twin birth is the same as what happens in a singleton birth. The three stages of labor are the same: the first stage during which the cervix dilates to 10 centimeters, the second stage when the babies are born, and the third stage when the placentas are born. You'll go through the first stage just once, as you would with a single baby.

You will however, have to go through the second stage twice. But the good news is that most women report they can rest for the 20 or 30 minutes that typically elapses between babies. And, because the cervix is completely dilated and stays that way for at least 30 minutes, there isn't usually any additional pain in delivering the second baby.

Your Recovery

For the first 24 hours after the babies were born I was kept in the labor and delivery area rather than sent back to my room, and monitored constantly by a nurse assigned only to me. It wasn't star treatment, believe me. It was because of the preeclampsia. At first, my liver function continued to decline and Dr. Ross told me later that my calcium levels were falling along with my platelet count, all of which means I remained very sick for the first day after the boys were born.

On the second day, my body began to stabilize, and they transferred me to the regular postpartum area, but I still couldn't eat. It's normal to be off food for a day or two after a cesarean, to allow your digestive system to begin working again after the shock of surgery. But for some reason, my system was quite slow to recover, and for four days I couldn't eat and I could drink very little. Of course I was receiving nutrients intravenously, but I was horrendously thirsty. Ice chips became my one desire; eating them the greatest thrill! I dreamt of them, vats and vats of ice chips. In those early days, before I could eat or drink, you could have offered me diamonds, champagne and caviar and I would have turned them all down for a cup of ice chips. Incidentally, being on a diet of ice chips alone, I lost a tremendous amount of weight in the hospital, but I wouldn't recommend that method!

After I was settled back in my room, I must have slept at some point, but my memory from the hospital is that I didn't sleep much. In fact it seemed the whole world started calling and sending flowers and visiting right away, and within a couple of days it did get to be too much. I was exhausted. Looking back at photographs, I look worse two or three days after the boys' birth than I did when I had preeclampsia and was undergoing a cesarean! If I had it to do over again, I would arrange to be more shielded from the excitement after the birth so that I could rest. You might want to consider arranging for that ahead of time. Of course there are always those people closest to us who we do want to include in such a momentous occasion, but we don't really have to share this time with *everyone* right away. I'd suggest making up a short list ahead of time, of those whom you want to come visit, and ask a friend to kindly keep others at bay for a few days at least.

To be honest, during those first days after a cesarean a big part of your awareness will be focused on the incision, which does hurt. But thankfully, there are very effective pain pills for that. When I took them, I felt little or no pain, and I didn't feel drugged. I was perfectly aware of everything and everybody around me, both emotionally and physically, and I was able to take care of the babies. Still, I had to fight my own silly instincts, which were to try to take fewer pain pills than were prescribed. If the doctor said I should have a pain pill every four hours, I'd try to stretch it to six hours. You and I know that's ridiculous, but it seems I do things like that because of some kind of crazy inner competition I engage in, along with the fact that I don't like being on medications of any kind. But after a day or so of that, even I could see that trying to minimize the number of pain pills I took only made me unnecessarily miserable. At the urgings of James and Dr. Ross I got back on schedule with the pain pills, and felt much better right away.

About 12 hours after the surgery, most obstetricians want you to get out of bed and move around a little. That wasn't something I looked forward to, but the nurses made it possible. They were fantastic in every way, from showing me how to brace the incision with my hands when I first stood up, to just being so kind and quick with an encouraging word. As much as we all appreciate a good doctor, when you're a patient in a hospital, the unsung heroes and heroines are the nurses. They make all the difference in your recovery, and I didn't meet a bad one while I was in the hospital. The shifts would change and I'd think "Oh, no. I really liked this one. I wish she wouldn't go." And then the new one would be even more wonderful than the one before.

The great thing about nurses on the maternity floor is that they can help you do what you so badly need to do after you've had these babies: they show you how to give something back to yourself. It is an incredible thing that happens when you get pregnant. From the day that you confirm your pregnancy every part of you, from your body to your spirit, belongs to these babies. Now for months it has been your responsibility to eat right for them, to exercise right for them, to not overwork for them, to stay calm for them. You've done whatever has been needed to be sure the babies would be healthy.

Once the babies are born, these wonderful nurses come and say, "It's your turn to be coddled. You should be proud of yourself. You did something amazing and we're here to help you take good care of yourself." My advice is to listen to them when they encourage you to take it easy, to rest, to be kind to yourself. Stay in the hospital as long as your insurance allows you to, and let these people care for you. Look at it this way: once you're home, how often will someone else be cooking your meals and doing your laundry for you, to say nothing of whisking a crying baby away so that you can sleep? Depending on what kind of help you have arranged for, that kind of care may happen for a short while, or it may never happen at all! And even if you do have help coming, there's a different mindset when you are home with babies. Ultimately, the responsibility for those babies falls squarely on your shoulders, help or no help, and that in itself can be exhausting and stressful. When you are in the hospital, you can still share the responsibility with the nurses. I wholeheartedly suggest you do that!

Before I'd had children, I assumed that the sooner I got back to my usual life the quicker my adjustment to having a baby would be complete. I've always been a high-energy, just-do-it kind of person, and I thought jumping back into the fray was the best way to get on with my life, even after a new baby. That's not really so. What I've learned from all my births is that if you rest well after having your babies, you'll regain your energy faster. I have a friend who said that after her first baby, she took off only a week or two before she was back out shopping for groceries and running errands, and she ended up really needing to nap every day for a year. With her next baby, she rested thoroughly for a month or more hardly going out at all, and arranged for friends to help her out during that time with all of the running around. Once she did go back to her normal life, she never felt draggy enough to need a nap.

For some of us, holding back and trying not to resume your pre-twins life right away is very difficult, but if you can do that, I truly believe you and your babies will reap the rewards, and will be more likely to enjoy life together. I hope that you'll start while you are still in the hospital, using that time to relax as much as possible. For me, that kind of relaxation had to happen at home. Not only did it seem that hundreds of calls came flooding through as soon as the babies were born, but within hours of the babies' birth, we noticed a person on the rooftop of the building across the street from the hospital. It was a photographer with a huge camera lens pointed in the direction of my room. We'd checked in under a false name to begin with, but when we spotted that camera, James lowered the blinds and called hospital admissions to change the name we were registered under. Still, the next day, he bumped into another photographer, this one he recognized from a major tabloid newspaper, walking down the hall and poking his

After the Birth

Whether you have a cesarean or a vaginal birth, in many ways your recovery should be similar to that of a woman who had one baby, with a few exceptions. Watch for:

- **Heavier postpartum bleeding.** Placental tissue— from one or two placentas—covered a larger area of your uterus, so there may be heavier bleeding. Tell your doctor if you are passing clots or if you think the bleeding is extremely heavy. It may mean some placental tissue is still in the uterus.
- **Possible anemia.** Because you may have heavy postpartum bleeding, and because the babies did challenge your iron stores anyway, you may become anemic after the birth. If you do, you'll likely feel dizzy and weak. Don't get out of bed without help, and talk with your doctor about iron supplements or ways to get more iron in your diet.

head into each room to find me! I don't know how the photographer managed to get onto the maternity wing but we knew our days in the hospital were numbered. At home it would be much easier to control who had access to me or to the babies.

In the days soon after the babies were born, I found that I was often close to tears over the smallest things. I wouldn't say that I was depressed, but I did feel very up-and-down emotionally. Sometimes I felt so grateful and in awe of the journey James and I had been on with these babies that the tears just overflowed. Other times I felt so touched by the babies and at the same time frightened for them. I felt as if I'd just climbed to the top of Everest to have them and now they faced a world fraught with possible trauma. Looking back, I think all that crying is quite normal,

---

- **Uterine cramping.** Your over-stretched uterus will take some time to shrink back to its normal size, and you may feel quite a bit of cramping as it does. It's part of the normal process that helps the uterus to settle back down into the pelvis. If you don't feel any cramping, which is more likely to happen after a multiple birth than after a single birth, it may be that there is some placental tissue retained in the uterus.

Let your doctor know immediately if you have a **fever,** which is a sign of infection, or if you have **pain on urination,** which is a sign of a bladder or kidney infection.

If you had a cesarean birth, watch for any **redness or swelling around the incision,** which may be a sign of infection.

If you had preeclampsia you may need to take blood pressure medication for a time after the birth, your blood pressure will be closely monitored, and you may have to stay in bed.

and as new mothers, we shouldn't be frightened of it. One of my friends said she cried unabashedly every day for at least six months after her babies were born, but she would never describe

---

What Is Postpartum Depression?

After your babies are born, various hormones make a quick tumble back to non-pregnant levels, and that can mean that you feel anything from a little more emotional to downright depressed. Everyone's sensitivity to hormonal changes is different, which is why some women feel these changes more acutely than others.

Keep in mind that you will also be dealing with change on a massive level after your babies are born, which is ample reason to feel overwhelmed or upset. Give yourself a break—don't expect yourself to handle everything without tears or the occasional meltdown. A few things you may be dealing with:

- One or both babies may have to remain in the hospital when you go home. Besides the sadness of not taking them both home with you, you may be worried about the health of one or both.
- Going home in itself may be scary.
- You will be exhausted at some point—maybe all the time for a while.
- You may not like the way you look now. You gained a lot of weight for the babies, and most of it is still there.
- You may have the "day-after-Christmas" blues. After all the build up to the birth, even with two wonderful, healthy babies in your arms everything may just seem anticlimactic.

herself as depressed. She felt that having the babies had opened her heart to a million joys as well as to a million sadnesses. There's so much poignancy in the fact of these little human miracles, who wouldn't cry at the thought of them?

Your Babies at Birth

I'd seen the boys for just a moment or two in the operating room, and then they were whisked away so quickly, I was left wondering where they were and what the medical team was doing with them. Thankfully, I had James there with me, to relay information from the doctors and nurses. He assured me the babies were fine, and he stayed with me for the 45 minutes or so it took for Dr. Ross to finish the surgery.

What Are They Doing with My Babies?

Here's what routinely happens right after each baby is born. Someone on each baby's medical team:

- clears the baby's airway.
- dries the baby and places her on a radiant warmer, an open crib or table with a heat source above.
- rates the baby on a scale of 1–10 according to the Apgar rating system, in which the baby's heart rate, respirations, muscle tone, reflexes and skin color are evaluated. Apgars are calculated at one minute and five minutes after birth.

They will also weigh and measure each baby, take her footprints, draw blood from a pinprick in her heel, give her an injection of vitamin K to aid in blood clotting, and administer eye drops to prevent eye infections.

As soon as they would let me go, one of the nurses wheeled me into the nursery. I was dying to get a really good look at each of the babies, and of course to get my hands on them. It's a good thing a nurse was with me, because I have to say that first glimpse of them was alarming. There was Kris, lying on his back, a tiny diaper taped around his middle, with his arms and legs splayed out to his sides. He looked limp, like a little doll that had been dropped. Wires crisscrossed his chest and ran to the edge of the warming bed. Covering at least half his body was a clear plastic tent, and through it I could see his tiny chest rapidly rising and falling, as if he'd just sprinted a mile. John lay on his own warming bed next to Kris, and his chest was also crossed by wires but there was no plastic tent over him. I was happy to see that he seemed to be cozily snuggled into a nest of receiving blankets. As I sat in my wheelchair beside him, Kris whimpered and cried out every few minutes, but John slumbered on, the epitome of mellow. That much was a comfort to me.

Mercifully, the nurse who had wheeled me in quickly began explaining the apparatus that surrounded my babies. Once again, knowledge proved to be my savior, and as the nurse spoke my discomfort at the sight of my babies dissolved. The plastic tent over Kris was called an oxyhood, and it gave him a little more oxygen than he had been getting when he was breathing room air. She told me he'd been working a little harder to breathe than they liked to see, and because he hadn't been getting quite enough oxygen, his skin color was what they called "dusky"—not quite blue, but not as pink as his brother. Now, under the hood, he was perfectly rosy.

John hadn't needed supplemental oxygen at all, and his Apgars had been a little higher than Kris's. The nurse pointed out to me that John's head was quite molded because it had been wedged deep in my pelvis. She showed me a tiny abrasion at the top of one of his ears that probably happened when Dr. Ross gently lifted him out—it must have been a tight squeeze!

The wires, she explained allowed the nurses to monitor all kinds of things about the babies, from each boy's body temperature, to his blood pressure, heart rate, and the amount of oxygen carried in his blood. It was comforting to know every aspect of their little bodies was being watched, but as I sat next to Kris and ran my fingers gently over his miniature fist, my heart ached to hold him.

Fortunately, Kris needed the oxygen only for the first day, and then he and John both graduated from the warming beds, each to his own enclosed incubator with two portholes in each side through which I could reach my hands to touch them. They were each still hooked up to a half-dozen monitors, but at least it was a little easier to get my hands on them. And I could open the incubators and take them out to hold them. Dr. Stern told us that neither Kris nor John was sucking very well, so they were both being fed formula through a tube placed in their noses, a method called *gavage* feeding. She assured me they'd be ready to suck in a few days, but it was hard to believe, watching them through the plastic walls that always seemed to separate us. I recall sitting between the two isolettes gazing at them each, and feeling sad not only that I couldn't hold them, but also sad for them, that they were so alone. They had spent all their lives to this point cuddled up with one another inside me, and now they each lived in their own little box. I know it was best for them, but I resolved then and there to try having them sleep in the same bed for a while when we got home, to give them back some of the comfort they must have felt with one another.

Even encased in plastic, wired for everything, I thought Kris and John were perfectly beautiful, completely gorgeous babies. However, when I look back at newborn photos of them, I have to admit that with their skinny little arms and legs and their relatively large heads, they looked like tiny versions of the movie character, ET. But I certainly didn't see them that way then. Doesn't it just seem to be part of a wonderful plan, how new mothers everywhere find their own babies to be infinitely fascinating and transcendently beautiful. If you've worried whether you'll like your babies once they are born, I hope you'll take comfort in this. You may feel panicked about caring for them, or frustrated when you can't get one to stop crying. But believe me, you'll look at your babies and then at everyone else's and you'll *know* without a doubt that yours are by far the cutest. That's Mother Nature at her best!

Your Family

Katie and Sean had been with me while I was in the hospital just before the babies were born, and I know that at 13 and 10 they were well aware of the fact that I was getting sicker and sicker before their eyes. Through that haze of illness, I remember my priority that day was to try to make sure they weren't frightened for me. I knew to some degree what I was going through was scary; just being hospitalized suddenly can be frightening. But I didn't want them to be overwhelmed by that feeling, so I really focused on how I was with them. I remained upbeat, confident, reassuring and certain that the babies and I were in good hands and right where we needed to be. That was the truth of course, and as it turned out focusing on my attitude for them served an additional purpose: I reassured myself, as well!

I was also aware that both Katie and Sean were incredibly excited about the babies, and about the fact that they were going to meet them soon. I was so grateful they had that attitude. Neither James nor I wanted them to feel they would be left out. It was a very big issue for us, and an important one for everyone who's having twins after having other children. The reality is that twins get so much recognition, just for being twins. They're instant superstars! First, as the mom, you get so much attention because you're carrying multiples. Then the babies come and they have center stage. James and I thought about it a great deal ahead of time. We decided that right from the time the boys were born, we would not only allow, but we'd encourage Katie and Sean to scrub up and go into the intensive care nursery to feed and hold Johnny and Kris. Anything the nurses would let them do was fine with us. Right away we could see that this had been the right decision. Katie and Sean couldn't get enough of holding the babies.

We remained on the lookout for ways to keep from instilling any fear in the older kids that they weren't grown up enough to deal with the babies. I wanted them to feel they were an important part of the babies' lives from the beginning, and that they were responsible enough to be.

Happily, the end result of Katie's and Sean's early experience helping to care for the babies has been that these babies are just about as much theirs as they are mine. At 14, Sean has a very special relationship with his 5-year-old brothers. They really look up to him; he's sort of their leader. And he loves to spend time with them. I don't think he minds being idolized by these little boys.

Katie, who was 13 when they were born, quickly became their little mom. She had been just starting to develop the dark side of teen life, sleeping a lot and being crabby when she was awake. But one look at these babies and she would just brighten up, so she couldn't manage to keep a really good teenage angst going. I began to have this strange feeling these boys were sent to our family to help us all, including our teenagers, gain perspective on life.

One more bonus to having teenagers around the babies was that Katie told me she realized immediately how much she loved looking after babies and what an incredibly satisfying feeling that was. At the same time, she also knew without a doubt how much she wouldn't want to do it for a long time yet in her own life. Without me ever having to say a word, she knew she didn't want to make a baby herself. She wanted her life and career first, but she knew she definitely wanted children at some point. And she knew that when she did have a child, the child would have to be the first priority in her life. It was fantastic watching her figure these things out and having her talk with me about what she had learned. Real life is a wonderful teacher—kids don't learn these kinds of things from books!

One of the many great sidelights about having twins is choosing their names. You get to use not one, but two of your favorite names; four if you're into middle names. In some families it can be a real group project just coming up with that many favorites. In our family it was just James and I who chose the names.

Actually, we settled on their names very quickly, early in the pregnancy. There was no searching and sifting through dozens of candidates. But strangely enough, the names they ended up with weren't exactly the ones we chose. We knew first of all that we wanted to name one John, after my father and after Johnny Cash, with whom we'd become good friends after he made several guest appearances on *Dr. Quinn.* We also knew we wanted the name Kristopher after my friend Christopher Reeve, but with a *K* instead of a *C* because we liked how that went with Keach.

That was all simple enough. The confusion came with the middle names. We had decided that Kristopher would have Stacy for a middle name, for James' father and brother, and that Johnny would have Steven for another friend, Steven Bickel. That way, each boy had a grandpa name. But it was not to be. *TV Guide* did an interview with me near the end of my pregnancy (the one for which Cheri had made me the beautiful dress I wore for the cover photo). When the story ran, which turned out to be less than a week before the boys were born, it included the boys' first names correctly, but switched their middle names. Immediately we began receiving gifts addressed to and engraved with the switched middle names, to John Stacy and Kristopher Steven. Before we knew it, the boys' *TV Guide* names were everywhere. To be honest, in the midst of giving birth and getting well afterward, as we hovered over the babies and adjusted to this new life with them, it no longer seemed that important to us which baby had which middle name. So we left the names the way *TV Guide* had published them.

You most likely won't have that kind of interference when you name your babies, but everyone seems to have a story about naming their twins. It *is* an important step in your babies' lives. If you have had a pregnancy like most women who have twins, you will have seen your babies via ultrasound many times before they are born. Like James and I, you may have also watched your babies' personalities evolve in utero, so you might have some idea which baby will be named what before they are born. I had thought I'd want to see them face to face before I decided which baby got which name. But as it turned out, the one we'd always called the mellow baby was the one nearest the incision, and as she lifted him into the world, Dr. Ross said, "There you are Johnny!" She was right—that one *is* Johnny—with the same crooked smile as my father, and the same placid nature.

So while certain aspects of naming your babies may be out of your control, I can only urge you to choose names that have meaning for you. But I would also urge you to think of the babies who will carry them, and of their circumstance as twins. Names that seem cute on infant twins can seem anything but cute on adults.

Of course while your babies are still tiny infants, almost any name may seem too big for them. You may find yourself doing what we did—using your own nicknames at first. Even after they were born, for the longest time we called the boys the names we'd had for them on the ultrasounds—This One and That One, as in, "I'll feed This One while you hold That One!"

The Straight Scoop:
Notes for Dads from James

What's the best thing I did during the boys' birth and the time immediately before and after? I stayed calm. That's what men can do for their wives. During the hours before the cesarean, I tried to be a calming influence as opposed to someone who creates anxiety even though inside, I was scared. I was scared I would lose Jane when Dr. Ross told me her condition was serious. But I didn't tell Jane about that conversation while it was all happening. Why tell her? I walked back into her hospital room and I said, "It's okay sweetie. Everything is going to be just fine."

When it was time for the cesarean, it was a little easier to be upbeat. I was ready; Jane was ready. "Let's go! Time to rock and roll," I told her. I wanted to say to Dr. Ross, "Give her the drugs, right away. Make her feel good! Pain isn't what I call a good experience." So I was relieved when the anesthesiologist gave Jane the epidural and saw that smile come on her face. I knew she could relax a bit.

After the babies are born, Dads, now is the time to realize it's not about you for a while. Mommy is all about the babies now. Still, you've been given this gift! Two babies! I hear guys grumble about not being able to be with their wives in the weeks after the birth. No sex. No privacy. Babies everywhere. It's like they want a reward for being given this amazing gift!

But guys, hang in there because there's nothing better than this. In a few years these tiny babies will be big. They'll be running around, giving you a kiss before going off to school. There's nothing better.

But say you've got a screaming baby in your arms right now, and you don't know what to do? Put him down in a safe place and leave the room for a few minutes. Take a deep breath. Love those babies anyway, whether they're screaming or not, and it all changes. They're crying this minute, smiling the next, and vice versa. You just have to go with it. Children are real teachers. They teach you about joy and being in the moment.

I believe that babies are the best luck you can have. They are good luck! They're not good luck in the sense that they're here to make you rich or famous. But they are in the sense that they offer you the opportunity to get out of yourself and think about someone else. I believe that most emotional pain comes from self-obsession, from thinking about Me all the time. Now you have these children and when you start thinking about them a little bit, you get immediately out of yourself.

That's the real gift.

Because I had been so ill, I was in the hospital with the boys for a full seven days. Barring complications, most women go home in about four days after a cesarean birth of twins, sooner after a healthy vaginal birth of twins. When I was finally ready to go home, leaving the hospital turned into a bit of a production because of the photographers who had been stalking us, apparently trying to get the first pictures of the boys. Luckily, there's a woman at Santa Monica Hospital, part of whose job it is to help deal with exactly this kind of situation. Her impersonations of well-known patients are quite believable.

On the day we were going home, she dressed up as me, sat in a wheelchair as they insist you do when you leave the hospital, borrowed a couple of babies and had someone wheel her out the front door of the hospital. I imagine the photographers who were lurking around were at least momentarily delighted, and then terribly disappointed!

While they fussed over her out front, James and I made our getaway, unseen, out the back way into a parking garage.

six

Taking Care of This One and That One

Taking care of your babies really starts when you are still in the hospital, but there you have those lovely nurses to help you out. And of course, every visitor is eager to hold a baby. In fact, between the nurses and friends and my other children, I could barely get my hands on my babies while I was still in the hospital. You may find that to be true, too, and like me, you may find that it's both a blessing and a bother. After they were born, although I was exhausted and really not well as a result of the preeclampsia, still, part of me longed to take over the boys' care completely, and tell everyone else to leave them to me!

The fact that Kris and John were in their little plastic incubators in the neonatal intensive care unit didn't help matters. Fortunately, that they were there at all wasn't a shock; we actually had been expecting they'd be there. Dr. Stern had explained before our boys were born that when any baby is born prematurely, the first few days of its life are usually spent in the NICU. The baby may be perfectly healthy, but a premature baby needs to be closely observed for a few days in order to be sure every part of him is in working order. She'd told us the same would be true for our twins if they were born before 37 weeks. And, if we had been expecting triplets or more, she told us we could plan that early or not, those babies would definitely have been in the NICU for a time.

So it was that our boys, who were basically healthy, were there for the first week of their lives. If your babies spend time in the NICU, you'll know what I mean when I say that it was hard to relate to them as babies when they had so many wires and monitors sprouting from everywhere. You cannot just scoop them up in your arms and love them. In order to hold either of them, monitors had to be adjusted or briefly disconnected, and the baby had to be positioned correctly in my arms to allow the monitor to be reconnected. During those first days of their lives, it felt to me like my boys were the nurses' patients rather than my babies.

Mercifully, neither Kris nor Johnny had any major health problems, and both came home from the hospital with me on December 7. I felt so lucky they could do that, but at the same time I felt sad for those mothers whose babies stayed behind when they went home. I was talking with one mother who'd been home for at least a week, and came to the hospital daily to be with her babies in the neonatal nursery. As we were leaving, I told her I was sorry her babies weren't home with her, and her response surprised me.

She shook her head and smiled. "Well, I do want them home eventually. But there's a bright side to everything," she said. "To tell you the truth, the babies are doing so well here that I'm not worried about them now. And in the meantime, I'm really catching up on my sleep! I'll be rested and ready for them when they've gained enough weight to come home."

I hadn't thought of it that way, but it just goes to show that so many times there is a silver lining to a situation, but we don't see it unless we can see life from the right angle.

What If My Babies Have to Stay in the Hospital When I Go Home?

Leaving your babies behind when you are discharged from the hospital is difficult for most new moms. Here are a few things you can do to help them, and yourself:

- Leave breast pads or stuffed animals you've slept with in each baby's isolette. Your scent will remind them of you.
- Make a tape recording of your voice speaking, or singing lullabies to be played in their isolettes. Premature babies are extremely sensitive to sounds, so be sure the volume is set very low.
- Pump milk for them to be fed until they are able to nurse. Studies have shown that mothers of premature babies have milk that is "specially formulated" by Mother Nature for the needs of their early babies. The hospital should have an electric pump you can use.

Feeding Your Babies

I had breast fed both Katie and Sean, and I loved every minute of it. But with the boys, I just wasn't sure I could do it. I was afraid I wouldn't be able to give them all the nutrition and the quantity of milk they needed, especially because they were so small, but also because I knew I would soon be working again. After I had become so ill just before they were born, I knew I really needed to concentrate on getting my own strength back. Those facts reaffirmed my decision to bottle feed instead of breast feed the babies.

Determined to be prepared, I had brought with me to the hospital an herbal tea that was supposed to keep my milk from coming in. For four days after the boys were born, I drank it daily. Late on the fourth day, one of the nurses came to me and said, "Now it's time for skin-to-skin contact with the babies."

"What do you mean?" I asked.

"That's when we undress each baby and put him on your chest, for bonding. It's good for you and for the baby," she explained.

I told her I was happy to have some time with the babies outside the isolettes, but I reminded her that I wasn't breast feeding. She nodded, said that was fine, and added that they'd only just begun to suck well enough to graduate from tube feeding to a bottle anyway.

With that assurance, she wheeled me off to the NICU. There she carefully lifted one of the boys from his isolette, complete with wires and monitors, took off the tiny t-shirt and diaper, and placed him on my bare chest. My mind was still a little foggy, and sadly, I don't remember which boy it was. But I do remember clearly that, even though he hadn't been able to suck for more than a day, that baby immediately started rooting—instinctively reaching his little mouth around to find my nipple.

Instantly, the enormously pleasurable feeling of nursing came flooding back to me.

"That's it," I thought. "There's no way I'm *not* going to breast feed!"

I stopped drinking the herb tea immediately, and, mercifully, it didn't have any effect on my milk supply. Within a day after the boys started nursing, my milk came in. It was the most wonderful feeling in the entire world—physically and emotionally—to feed those babies myself. The babies each just latched right on, and it was total joy for me. There was joy in knowing they were getting the unique immunities and nutrients that come only from human milk. And there was a softer, deeper joy I felt when all three of us snuggled together as they nursed. My sweetest memories of their newborn days, in fact, are of nursing them both at once, with the monitors hidden out of the way. When they were in my arms, and I was feeding them it finally felt like they were my babies.

Will My Babies Be Able to Nurse If They Are Premature?

If your babies are born at a full 34 weeks' gestation or later, they will most likely be able to suck well enough to either nurse or to take a bottle. If they are born right at 34 weeks or earlier, they may have not yet developed the ability to suck effectively. In that case they may be fed by *gavage,* in which a tiny tube is inserted into the nose or mouth and threaded down to the stomach. A vial of formula or breast milk attached to the tube slowly flows into your baby's stomach. Very early babies who cannot yet be fed by gavage can be given nutrients intravenously, which is called *parenteral nutrition.* Some babies are fed using a combination of these methods.

If your babies are fed in these ways, talk with your doctor about when each baby is likely to develop the ability to suck. At that time, you can begin nursing or bottle feeding. While you are waiting for your babies to be able to breast feed you can keep your milk supply up by using an electric breast pump. The hospital or a local chapter of La Leche League (a breast feeding support group) should be able to loan or rent one to you inexpensively.

Once I started nursing, I felt really bad, extremely guilty that I'd even considered *not* breast feeding. Again, it was the nurses who came to my rescue and helped me sort out those feelings. They reminded me that bottle feeding is a perfectly legitimate choice, particularly given the fact that I did have other children and a husband to deal with, and a career I knew I was going back to. They also reminded me that breast feeding doesn't go smoothly for everyone and that if I didn't feel comfortable about it, even now, I shouldn't do it.

Best of all, the nurses made me feel good about the fact that I could feed the babies myself as much as I was able to, and that formula would take care of the rest of their feedings. They assured me that in spite of everything—health, family, and career—it was entirely possible, even for someone like me to breast feed these babies. Suddenly I understood that the breast-or-formula decision was not an either/or proposition, and that gave me confidence. The babies had taken bottles already, so I knew it wouldn't be a huge problem for them to move from bottle to breast and back again if we needed to. What a relief that was, to know I didn't have to feel traumatized, stressed or worried about them getting enough nutrition exclusively from me. I could really relax into nursing them. Knowing all of this was very freeing to me, and if you're struggling with this decision, I hope it will be for you, too.

As it turned out I didn't use formula at all for nearly eight weeks. I fed them entirely on breast milk for that time, and after that, on a combination of breast milk and formula. Believe me, there was plenty to go around!

Nursing meant I had to drink what seemed like gallons of water each day, and once again, I had to eat almost constantly to keep my own system going and to feed those babies. I ate as nutritiously as possible and I avoided coffee, alcohol, chocolate, and spicy foods. Thai food didn't sit particularly well with the babies, but I love it, so occasionally I'd cheat and have a tiny taste of it anyway, and I'd usually get away with it. My babies seemed to do fine with other foods, but I quickly found from talking with girl-friends that every one of us was carefully avoiding certain foods—and that the foods we avoided were all different. What you can eat, and what you cannot, depends for the most part on the baby, and on what his or her digestive system can handle. For some moms that meant no broccoli; for others it meant staying away from dairy products or from tomatoes. We each figured these

How Can I Be Sure I Have Enough Milk for Two Babies?

Nursing is the ultimate example of supply equaling the demand. In other words, the amount of milk you have is primarily dependent upon how much the baby sucks. A baby sucking at the breast stimulates production of the hormone oxytocin, which in turn stimulates the production of milk. Of course you need to be eating well and drinking plenty of water. But if you do, and you also let your babies nurse as frequently as they want to— and they will want to be fed more often than formula fed babies because human milk is digested more efficiently—your body will produce the amount of milk they need.

You'll know your babies are getting enough milk if they each:

- soak at least six diapers a day, and they each have at least one bowel movement in each 24-hour period.
- gain an average of one-half to one ounce per day during the first two to three months after they come home from the hospital.

If your babies are not doing either of these, check with your pediatrician right away.

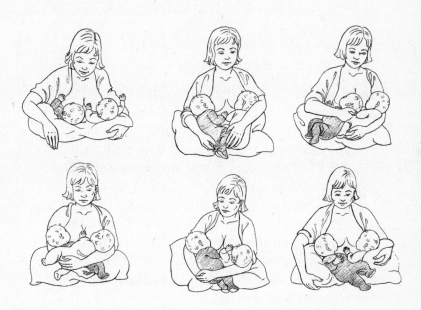

Some breast feeding positions you might want to try.

things out through trial and error and by paying attention to how our babies acted after they were fed, as well as by keeping track of what we'd eaten earlier in the day. Fortunately, as our babies grew, we found that they all became generally less sensitive to what we'd had to eat.

How Much Should I Eat While I'm Breast Feeding?

You'll need to eat 1,000 to 1,200 additional calories a day to breast feed two babies. It takes about 2,000 calories daily to support the normal weight of an average-sized woman, which is considered to be about 5'5". That means if you are of average size, you will need to eat 3,000 to 3,200 high-quality calories each day.

Keep in mind that studies have shown the nutrient content of breast milk remains fairly constant no matter what the mother's diet is like. Not eating well, or enough, will have an effect on *your* body and on how *you* feel.

Most nursing mothers are also extraordinarily thirsty. When you were pregnant, your doctor most likely advised that you drink at least eight 16-ounce glasses of water a day. You'll still need at least that much and probably more, although now it may be easier to consume. Extreme thirst provides great motivation!

It may seem like it's forever that you have to avoid certain foods and be careful about your diet, but really it's only for a couple of months, and they fly by faster than you'd ever imagine. Plus, there are more bonuses for you as a mom than just the satisfaction and the pleasurable feeling of nursing—although those are pretty important bonuses in my opinion. First of all, I thought it was just simpler to pick up a baby and feed him than to always be preparing bottles. Even with the pumping, nursing never seemed like that big of a hassle.

Another plus is that with the calorie drain that nursing babies produce, you will likely lose quite a bit of your baby weight over the next few months without having to diet—which is of course against the rules anyway while you're nursing. However, you probably won't lose all of that extra weight as long as you are nursing. Everyone's different, but I know that many women find their bodies seem to want to hold on to a certain amount of baby weight while they're breast feeding, presumably as nutritional insurance for the mother as well as for the baby. I know I had a slightly pouchy abdomen until I completely stopped nursing, which was when the boys were about three months old.

Another important plus I found was that nursing the boys required that I sit down and rest. As seems to be typical of people like me with type A personalities, after the boys were born and I started feeling better I had the hardest time making myself slow down and rest so that I wouldn't become totally exhausted. But every time the babies needed to nurse, which of course happened every couple of hours at the beginning, I had to sit down, snuggle up with them, and put my feet up. Nothing else in the world could have made me do that so regularly as feeding my boys.

When the boys were still newborns, I also found that with breast feeding I didn't have to make such a big deal about who had eaten what and at what time. I usually nursed them together, and I just made sure to switch the babies' positions each time I fed them to help my milk supply develop evenly on each side, and remain that way. At first I did keep a little notepad with me to help me keep track, but soon it became second nature. For example, if Johnny had nursed on the right and Kris on the left at mid-morning, I'd be sure at the next feeding that Johnny nursed on the left and Kris on the right.

Of course the most obvious bonus every nursing mother enjoys is larger breasts. I must say mine became huge when my milk came in. It was pretty much a stunner, but I always had a sense of humor about it. For a while there I looked like I had two huge footballs on my chest. Even if you're not partial to large breasts, remember that when they are so much bigger, the rest of your body looks smaller! So if you can somehow tuck your tummy muscles in, you're liable

What If I Want to Bottle Feed?

The most important issue concerning how you feed your babies is that you feel comfortable and confident about whatever decision you make.

Many hospitals give out cow's-milk-based formulas. If your babies have trouble with this type of formula, (and they'll let you know with their excessive spitting up, diarrhea, gasiness, fussiness, and/or diaper rashes) you can talk to your doctor about other options, such as soy or protein-hydrolysate formulas. Even if only one of your babies has a problem with a specific formula, save your sanity by talking to your doctor about switching both babies to the same formula.

Formula comes in three forms: ready-to-use liquid which is convenient but expensive, liquid concentrate that must be mixed with sterilized water, and powder which also must be mixed carefully with sterilized water to avoid lumps. You can **fill and refrigerate bottles the night before** to help you stay ahead of your babies' feeding needs, and you may want to **color-code bottles to each baby** so you can more easily keep track of who has taken how much formula. Then gently warm the bottles in a bowl of hot tap water until a drop on the inside of your wrist feels warm, not hot.

to look like you're in pretty good shape for someone who just had twins. Besides, those nursing breasts are a great distraction from other parts of your body that may not be back in the shape you'd like for quite a while yet. I suggest you dress accordingly and enjoy those large breasts while you have them!

As soon as we got home from the hospital with the babies, I became very familiar not only with the big electric breast pump we had on loan from the hospital, but also with a smaller portable pump that seemed to go with me everywhere. It wasn't just that I always seemed to be stockpiling milk for night feedings that someone else could give the babies. It was that my breasts would get over-full if I was out at a time when I might normally be feeding the boys, and it could feel like an explosion was imminent if I didn't pump away some of the excess. So no matter where I was, I knew when it was pumping time, just like clockwork. I wasn't often out at feeding time, but if I was caught while I was out shopping, I'd find a clean, quiet ladies' lounge. At dinner parties, I'd go up into someone's bedroom. There was an unforgettable moment in the home of a very famous, major figure in the film industry whose elegant wife had never had children. Poor man came home from work one evening and there I was in this extremely fancy bathroom area pumping away. I thought to myself afterwards—could that be why I've never seen those people since? At the very least, he probably never again thought of me as a glamorous actress!

Going Home/Getting Help

On the day before we were set to go home from the hospital with the boys, Dr. Stern was examining them when, listening to him through her stethoscope, she noticed that Johnny had a little bit of a heart murmur. She didn't think it was serious, but just in case, we set up an appointment with a cardiologist for the next day. After examining Johnny, the cardiologist agreed that it wasn't anything to be concerned about, but I can tell you that my own heart was doing flips as we waited for his diagnosis.

There is no worry like the worry a parent can feel for the well-being of her child, and James and I were enormously relieved that Johnny was fine. Still, I felt like we needed to keep our eyes glued to him and his brother, as if that would prevent anything and everything bad from happening to them. Even as an experienced mother, I felt concerned when we went home, and found myself not wanting them to leave my sight. And that can be exhausting! I believe that you simply must have another pair of eyes and hands to help you in the beginning, until you become experienced enough to relax a little with your babies. Without all the help I had, I really don't think I could have survived those first weeks alone with the babies, wonderful as they were.

No matter what your situation, whether you are going back to work or not, every mother of twins deserves to have some regularly scheduled help—paid or not—at home for at least the first month after the babies are born. I know there are a few super moms who really don't want help with their babies and who really don't need it. But for me, and maybe for you, having help can contribute enormously to both your sanity and your energy levels. You do have a responsibility to yourself and your family to get your own strength back, and letting someone else take up the slack will help you do that. Eventually, of course, you will have to learn how to take care of the babies on your own. But I firmly believe that having help in the beginning gives you a chance to develop a workable home routine under less stressful circumstances than if you were all alone with the babies all the time.

Perhaps you've already arranged to have help at home. Good for you! But perhaps you haven't, or maybe you don't have a plan for help because you think you can't afford it. If either of these sound like you, I want to tell you two things: First, it's not too late to get help. Second, there's always a way, no matter what your family budget.

Staying in the hospital for as long as your insurance will allow is a good start. You'll have days during which those wonderful nurses can give you lots of baby care tips if you ask them, and they will let you practice your new baby care skills, easing you into taking care of two babies by yourself. If I were you, I'd also keep a list of visiting friends who might be able to help out once you're home. If that seems like too much to think about when you are still tired from the birth, ask a friend or your husband to make that list for you.

Once you are home with your babies, choose a couple of friends from your list and ask them to visit you on a regular basis as their schedules allow, maybe just one afternoon a week each. When you have two newborns, simply having a friend join you in your kitchen for tea (which she makes for you) and holding a baby or two can be heaven. Or, perhaps your friend could hold down the fort for half an hour while you go out for a walk, or drive to the mall to window shop (*not* to run errands—ask another friend to do those for you!). Maybe she could help you fold laundry while you catch up on local gossip.

This is a time when the smallest indulgences can seem like the greatest gifts. I found that two things in particular became so precious in the weeks after the boys were born: time alone and adult contact. I loved the babies dearly, but honestly, when you're home all day with them, you do begin to wonder if you are capable of a coherent thought. It seems your mind is taken up with thoughts only of the next feeding or the next diaper change. A little chat with a girlfriend can go a long way toward making you feel like you're still a part of the larger world. And to get some time alone—that too can be a slice of heaven. I have a girlfriend who told me her greatest joy when her twins were infants was to go to the grocery store alone, not to buy groceries for her family, but to read the magazines, uninterrupted. One's standards do change with the arrival of twins!

James also helped out immensely, and I hope that like James, your husband will consider himself a full partner in this project. If you are breast feeding and supplementing with bottles, your husband can feed the babies sometimes, either with breast milk you have pumped or with formula. Perhaps he could take one middle-of-the-night feeding so you can sleep, especially if he has maternity leave from his work (which some companies do give fathers these days) and he won't have to get up the next morning. If that's not the case, he could bring a hungry baby (or two) to you in bed so that you can nurse there without having to get up or even to wake up completely.

Aside from family and friends, there are other places to look for unpaid help, or help that won't charge you too much. I know families who have had great success calling on church groups, Girl Scout troops, high school child care or community service classes, or YMCA babysitting classes. The helpers get much-needed experience, and the mom gets a break. With younger helpers of course you may not be able to leave your babies alone with them, but it is still a joy to have someone take even a little of the load off your shoulders. And, don't be shy about asking your helpers to do something other than take care of the babies. Ask them to run errands, mow the lawn, start dinner, or to do other such chores while you spend time playing with the babies. Too often we women rush around doing all the work, while the baby-sitter is home having playtime with the kids. You deserve to have fun with your babies too!

The other option, of course, is to pay for professional help. It is extraordinarily expensive to hire a baby nurse or two, but I have to say that if you can swing it financially, it is an enormous relief to have them. Even if the expense seems frightening to you, I hope you'll keep in mind there may be more ways than one to pay for a baby nurse. I found that friends were constantly asking me what kind of gifts I wanted for the babies, and I imagine people are asking you the same thing. Why not tell them you want a gift certificate that you can use toward paying a baby nurse?

James and I arranged far in advance of the babies' birth with a local agency for full time, 24-hour help. The agency we used was one recommended by friends, but you can find one in your area by looking in the phone book under Child Care or a similar heading. We booked two baby nurses to work 12 hours each—a day nurse and a night nurse. If you're thinking that one nurse would be all your budget could handle, I would suggest getting a night nurse, so that you will be able to sleep through the night whether or not your babies do. You can, like I did, pump milk during the day for the babies to be fed at night. The sure promise that you'll get a decent night's sleep may in itself be worth the cost of the nurse, and it can make the days a little easier!

We'd arranged for the nurses to come just after we *thought* we were going to have the babies, which was December 20. However, because the boys arrived early, on November 30, all our planning was for naught. If that happens to you, rest easy. We quickly found that once you have one baby nurse, she'll likely know someone else she can recommend. The nurses we'd booked were still on other jobs when we needed them, but through their baby nurse network, we found other baby nurses pretty easily.

Even though it was terribly expensive, in our case the two nurses were incredibly necessary. When we went home from the hospital, I was still trying to get my health and energy back, as well as feed the babies. Because of my health, for me to get up in the middle of the night and lose sleep doing so wasn't going to work. On top of all that, within two months I knew I would be going back to *Dr. Quinn,* and getting up at 5:00 or 6:00 in the morning to go to the set. My being able to sleep at night—as well as work during the day—and have the babies well cared for were all necessities. So our baby nurses really were a godsend. They each did all the necessary work with the babies, but when I wanted to bathe the boys, or when it was time for me to feed them, I would jump right in. Plus, I had the peace of mind of knowing that the nurses were watching the babies like hawks, night and day, and that they were experienced professionals. I really felt so grateful for them and how much they helped us in the transition from a family with teenagers to a family with teenagers *and* babies. I swear, if I had a magic wand, I'd grant every family with newborn twins a month of baby nurse care!

If you're not convinced you need outside help because you have older children, I believe they are precisely why you might reconsider employing someone at least for a while. I found that having dependable help with the babies meant that I was able to be there for my other children so that they didn't feel so pushed out of the picture. When Katie and Sean came home from school in the afternoon, I didn't want to have to hush them or have them wait for me forever because I was dealing with the babies. They were both so great with the babies anyway, they did eventually become another wonderful source of help. But before that, we were all able to ease into our roles because we could rely on the baby nurses to take care of the difficult tasks. Meanwhile, Katie and Sean really got to know the babies first by just playing with them. They both loved to feed them if I'd expressed milk, and they loved just to hold the babies, to rock them to sleep. I'll admit they weren't as wild about changing the babies' diapers, but they did change them sometimes. One of my favorite moments was to find Katie or Sean—or both of them—curled up with a baby or two, asleep on the couch in the babies' room.

I felt it was as important for the older kids to bond with them as it was for James and myself, and it was such a treat to watch them as they did. The more love you can give your babies—not just from one person, but from everyone around them—the better.

Bumps in the Road

Coming home from the hospital with the babies was an enormous event for us. Everyone who hadn't seen the babies in the hospital wanted to see them now. My sisters and mother were visiting from England, as well. So within days of bringing the babies home, we had a big reception so everyone, friends and family, could come at one time to welcome the boys. Kris and Johnny were passed around quite a bit that evening, probably too much, as it happened. The first sign that it was all too much for them was when my sister Sally was holding Johnny. The baby nurse, who was peering over Sally's shoulder, suddenly saw that Johnny was turning blue. She grabbed him from Sally, and the gentle jostling of being handed from one person to the other seemed to stimulate him to take a deep breath or two. Quickly, the blue tinge to his skin disappeared, and he was his usual rosy pink again. I was across the room at the time, so I didn't know anything had happened. But about half an hour later, the nurse was standing next to me and holding Johnny. This time I saw him begin to go blue, and I was terrified.

The jostling worked again as I grabbed him from her arms, and even though he was pink again, I was on the telephone to the pediatrician in an instant. Dr. Stern told us to bring both boys in right away. We had only been home for four days, and already here we were, heading back to the hospital. It was disappointing, but I was too terrified to worry much about that.

Johnny seemed fine during the car ride there, but I couldn't take my eyes off him for a second; I watched every breath. Once we were there, it was actually comforting to be back at the hospital where I knew he'd have help immediately if he needed it. Still, this visit proved to be especially exhausting. I was up all night nursing Johnny while he was on a special monitor to track his breathing and his heart rate. Meanwhile, after examining him, Dr. Stern said that Kris seemed fine. He actually slept through it all and I pumped some milk for him in case I was preoccupied with Johnny when he awoke.

The next day, Dr. Stern tested both twins further for apnea and bradycardia (see box on page 156), as well as for various respiratory infections that can cause them. The tests showed the boys were healthy, and that only Johnny had both conditions. Still, when we went home later that day, it was with two monitors, just in case Kris developed the same thing. Each baby had his own gray control box with two wires leading from it that ended in little adhesive monitor pads, like tiny round Band-Aids, which we stuck onto their chests.

While we knew it was a good thing to have those monitors, they just about drove us all crazy. It seemed the alarm on one monitor or the other was going off all the time; I think we had at least 10 false alarms for every real one. A dislodged adhesive pad, a poor connection between the pad and the baby's skin, or just a normal change in the baby's breathing could set one of them off. But Dr. Stern told us that if an alarm did go off, within 30 seconds someone should be rubbing the baby's back to get him to breathe again. So whenever there was a peep out of the machine, at least three people in our

What Is Apnea?

Apnea is the absence of breathing for 15 seconds or more, and is fairly common in premature babies. Nearly half of babies who weigh less than 5½ pounds at birth have apnea spells in the first few weeks of life, as do about 85 percent of those weighing less than 2½ pounds. It's often accompanied by bradycardia, or slowing of the heart rate. Both are thought to occur because the centers in the brain that control respiration are not yet mature. Some babies may also have episodes of apnea if they are too hot or cold, if they are stressed or fatigued, or even during normal feeding and handling.

Occasionally babies can pull out of an apnea episode themselves, especially if the baby is on a monitor and the alarm goes off, reminding the baby to breathe. But in more serious forms of apnea, breathing does not resume, and the baby becomes a dusky blue-gray color because of lack of oxygen. Gently rubbing the baby's back, arms or legs usually is enough to revive the baby. If it does not, the baby can be given extra puffs of room air through a procedure called bagging, or the baby may be given oxygen.

For most babies, periods of apnea disappear within a few days or weeks. For others it may take months for the apnea to resolve, and these babies may be at home with a monitor which tracks heart and breathing rates.

household, (usually James, myself, and one of the baby nurses) would run to wherever the babies were. It was nerve wracking because you'd never know which alarm was the real thing. Like the burglar alarm that you don't dare ignore because you don't know if it was the cat walking in the door that triggered it or not, we treated all of the monitor's alarms as if they were real emergencies. We also knew that someone always needed to be paying attention to the babies' skin color too. We reasoned that if the monitor gave us so many false positives, couldn't it also give us false negatives? That was yet another reason to be especially thankful for the night nurse. As we slept, I could feel confident that someone was sitting next to the babies' beds, literally staring at them all night long.

The second time we came home from the hospital we made sure our homecoming was a quiet one. No big receptions, no stress for the babies. We all needed a little time and a lot more peace to recuperate from our early bumps in the road.

Back to Work

In all, I was away from *Dr. Quinn* for about a month before the boys were born, and for another six weeks after they were born. In mid-January we were scheduled to begin shooting again. But my return to work was different from what most mothers experience when they go back to work—my babies came with me. For that, I feel especially blessed.

On the set, I had my trailer as always, but now, right next to it, there was also a trailer for the babies. It was outfitted with cribs, changing tables, toys, a small kitchen—everything we needed to set up a miniature household. Each day, after their morning routine at home, the baby nurse would bring them out to the set, which meant that from the moment I returned to work, the babies were with me almost all day, every day. When they were very small, between scenes I'd run back to the baby trailer every available minute and feed them, or pump for them.

Pumping continued to be a way of life for me. Poor Kelly, my hairdresser. This unmarried man who hadn't, I'm sure, given a single thought to pregnancy and babies until I came along, continued to have quite an education in both subjects. Not only had he been there to watch me throwing up repeatedly and uncontrollably when I was pregnant, he also got to watch Lesa my makeup artist who got pregnant a couple of months after me, throwing up in the same trailer.

The timing wasn't a coincidence. Lesa and her husband had been wanting to start a family, and she timed her pregnancy to happen with mine, so we'd both have the same maternity leave. Lesa had her son Luke soon after the boys were born, and Luke joined Johnny and Kris in the baby trailer. The three boys became best friends immediately. Once Luke joined us, Kelly got to listen to both Lesa and I as we pumped milk for our babies. Each morning, he was treated to the sound of our electric breast pumps whirring away, and the sight of us each hooked up to our own pumps. One or the other of us also often had to sneak off to pump in the middle of shooting as well. We'd rehearse a scene and then if Lesa or I—or both of us—had become over-full we would have to literally run back to my trailer to pump. It was really a bizarre sight, and we began to laughingly call my trailer the dairy barn. Cheri made certain my costumes during that period were easily opened in the front, so I could accommodate all the pumping and nursing.

The funniest part was that when we returned to shooting after the boys were born, I was playing Michaela Quinn about seven or eight months pregnant, and I was wearing this huge pregnancy pad. I was pretty proud of the fact that I'd lost my baby weight, but no one on the set ever got to see evidence of that because I was wearing that pregnancy pad every day. Even though it was uncomfortable at times, and a little annoying to be walking around looking pregnant when I'd just finished with that myself, I must say that when I had the babies with me, they fit really nicely, balanced on top of that pad. It was a perfect little shelf for one or both babies to sit upon.

Coming to Terms

Babies change one's life in more far-reaching ways than anything else can. When you have two babies, the change is that much greater. And when you have two babies about whose health you are even a little bit worried, it can disorient you so much you feel you don't know which end is up any more.

James and I felt that way after our return to the hospital with the boys. In the quiet days we spent at home following that episode, we talked about how frightening Johnny's breathing problems had been and how surreal it was when it happened. In a way, we couldn't believe this was happening to Johnny; to us. James said he felt it was as if a whirlwind had picked us up, and had plunked us down in a strange baby-land filled with wondrous sights, but terribly frightening ones too, as well as so many things we didn't understand.

Of course everything turned out fine for us and for Johnny, but it gave us an unforgettable taste of what it is like for many parents of twins. If you are struggling with all the feelings and fears that surround having one or two babies who are not well, I can only tell you what worked for us in the short time we were where you are. James and I found great comfort in depending on one another. When I'm over-emotional he's generally calm, and the solidity I feel from him calms me in turn. That may not be exactly what your marriage is like, but that doesn't matter. What matters is that you look first to one another for strength in areas where you may lack strength yourself. Your marriage will be the better for it, and your babies will benefit from that too.

I'd also urge you to look to others to get the information you need about your babies' difficulties. We found the NICU nurses to be unfailingly helpful and compassionate. After our experience with Johnny's breathing problems, the fear I felt at first really all but disappeared when I understood what caused his apnea and how we could deal with it. It was almost like learning a new language to understand it all, but knowing what the nurses and Dr. Stern were talking about made everything not only more familiar, but also less threatening.

Looking back on the pregnancy and the boys' birth, I'm struck by the mind-boggling array of lessons to be learned from the experience. Perhaps one of the biggest lessons for me was that

I had the opportunity to gain a greater understanding of what I could control and what I could not. In our many failed attempts to get pregnant, James and I both did everything in our power to create the environment that would produce a pregnancy, and then we had to sit back and take what came—and it wasn't always what we'd wanted so badly. The same was true again when the boys were born. And again when we returned to the hospital with them. Now I see that each was a distinct opportunity to understand how little control we really have over the outcome of things!

That basic lack of control over the outcome of things we do, or over things our children do means to me that it takes great faith to have children, and to raise them. Faith that we will learn as we go along, faith in our ability to live with a heart that's newly tender with love for these babies, and faith that we can bear to harbor that tiny spark of fear we hold for the well-being of those dearest to us. Having the faith to take a deep breath, open our eyes, and plunge ahead caring for our babies with all the confidence we can muster, as if we knew what we were doing—now that's a real gift.

I hope you'll be patient with yourself and with each other as you learn how to handle that gift, and the precious cargo you now hold in your arms.

seven

Feathering a Nest for Two Babies

Almost every woman I know goes through a period of nesting before her baby comes. In my earlier pregnancies, I would usually do the most obvious thing: I'd get into some kind of cleaning mood, scrubbing out sinks and polishing tile in the bathroom, sweeping out the garage. Every time I've had a baby I've become a clean freak. In fact I have a photograph of me the day before I had Katie, sweeping out a bathroom.

Not everyone cleans in preparation for childbirth. I know one woman who could always tell when the birth was near by her urge to clear out closets, tossing out old sweaters and galoshes and whatever else she found, often much to her husband's chagrin. Another friend couldn't resist painting the trim in her babies' room, bending and reaching all day until she was exhausted. Then, just as she was telling her husband, between yawns, that she really needed a good night's sleep, her water broke. No sleep for her that night!

With my boys, I could tell I was really nesting when, at eight months pregnant I seriously considered climbing a ladder in order to hang the stuffed animals on the wall mural in their room. Fortunately, I came to my senses before I put my foot on the bottom rung, but there was no question I simply had the itch to do *something* to make me feel I was really getting ready for the babies.

Cleaning and rearranging things may be satisfying, but I've come to believe that when you're pregnant with twins, the safest nesting activity is to start collecting the clothing and equipment you'll need for your babies. It's something you can do even if you're on bed rest. Put your feet up and thumb through some of the great baby gear catalogues available now. Once you're surrounded by all those new (or borrowed) baby things I can almost guarantee you'll begin to feel truly prepared!

From my own experience, there are a few rules of thumb to follow as you feather the nest for your twins. First, because you will have two babies to dress, to bathe, to care for, *everything* you buy should be the utmost in simplicity and function. It may also be lovely to look at, or cute to wear, but for you, function must come first. As a mother of twins, you will have more than enough to do, so make sure that whatever you buy really *works* for you before it has a place in your life. Watch for things that can be operated or used with one hand (such as a tube of diaper ointment with a flip top instead of a twist-off top). Get in touch with other twin moms through your local twins clubs or your childbirth preparation class, and talk with them about best buys. As a mother, I feel that I am constantly learning about and refining how I care for my children. I also find—and I think you will too— that most other moms are quite generous about sharing what they've learned.

My second rule of thumb is that you don't always need two of everything. Of course you need two snowsuits, but you don't really need two baby baths. My philosophy is the fewer accessories you have to deal with, the better, and with two babies, you'll have plenty no matter what.

Last, I believe in trying out big items before I buy them, if it's at all possible. For example, my boys loved being in the Snugli carrier. But I know of people whose babies howled whenever they were in it, and others who found that "wearing" two babies for even a short time gave them such an aching back they couldn't imagine putting on the contraption again after their first time. I'd suggest that you either wait until after your babies are born, then borrow an item like this in order to try it first, or that you buy it from a store that will let you return it.

Dressing Your Babies

If you're trying to economize, here's one place where you can have your cake and eat it too. Everyone you know will give you dozens of perfectly adorable outfits for your babies, so you don't have to buy them. But no one is likely to give you the basic layette—you know, the practical things like undershirts and pajamas. So I say, let everyone give you the lovely, pricey outfits, while you save your money for the everyday items, which are much less expensive. And you may be able to find extra savings in that area. Some stores specializing in baby clothing may give you two-for-one prices on basic layette items if you tell them you have twins. Not every store is going to be willing to do this, especially with so many twins being born now, but it's worth asking for a twin discount.

When you're buying your babies' clothing, be careful about sizes. Right after our boys were born we realized that all the clothing we had already bought was standard newborn size, and far too big for them. In a panic attack we rushed out and bought all these preemie-sized clothes. Needless to say they grew out of those really fast—in a matter of a few weeks. And on top of that, we quickly saw that we'd bought far too many tiny things as well. All the boys really wore, out of the huge selection of clothing we had bought, was about a half-dozen undershirts and some pajamas, just like they had in the hospital. The rest of the clothing was barely worn, if it was worn at all. So we cleaned all those tiny things beautifully, pressed them and took them all to the intensive care nurses to give to other babies and their families.

Once Kris and Johnny grew out of their preemie clothing, I found that whatever size I bought, it was better that it be a little large rather than a little small. The boys seemed more comfortable, and it was easier to get the clothing on and off of them. And of course, they would eventually grow into it anyway.

The first size after preemie size is newborn, which usually translates to size 3-6 months. Depending on how big your babies are at birth and on how fast they grow, you might skip newborn size altogether. Generally speaking, I think it's frustrating at first to figure out what size your babies will wear, because it seems there just isn't a standard size baby. Johnny and Kris are perfect examples of that. They were born early and weighed four and four and a half pounds at birth, but by they time they were six months old, they were about 17 and 18 pounds. I have friends whose full-term twins didn't weigh that much until they were nearly a year old! So in choosing clothing, I always looked for labels that specified a weight to go with the size, because I could choose pretty accurately then. If you can't find those, talk to a knowledgeable salesperson in the baby department. The good news is that once you do figure out

How Much Clothing Will I Need for Two Newborns?

Because of spitting up and diaper leaks, you can plan on about four complete clothing changes a day for each baby. You can decide how many sets of clothing you need based on how often you want to do laundry, and whether you have a washing machine at home or you'll be going to a laundromat. You probably won't want to go there more than twice a week, and if you're doing laundry at home, you will most likely do laundry about every other day. Given that kind of a plan, for basic clothing such as undershirts and pajama-type play-suits, about eight to 12 of each should be enough.

how your babies' age and weight translate to clothing sizes, you've got a pattern you can usually follow for a long time. Until then, it seems it's just trial and error. Which is all the more reason to buy only a few things at first and see how they fit, so you won't find yourself either storing dozens of useless outfits, or making lots of trips to the store to return items.

Everything I bought for the boys to wear, I bought in the softest fabric imaginable, and I always ran my hands inside and out to see if there were rough seams or little decorations that might bother them. I love the feel and the breathability of 100 percent cotton, and used that whenever I could, except in sleepwear which must be specially treated to be fire resistant.

My favorite simple outfit for the boys when they were infants was a little one-piece T-shirt that snaps at the crotch, to be worn over the diaper. Short sleeved and in solid colors or charming prints, they made a nice tidy outfit the boys could wear for play in warm weather. The shirt has a wide neck and generous arm openings so that it was easy to dress even wiggly baby boys. Just be sure any clothing you get for your babies comes with snaps, not buttons. Baby buttons are far too tiny. They were such a struggle for me to button and then just when I'd finished sliding each one through the equally tiny slit of a buttonhole, the darned things would slide right out again. Worse, buttons can come off, and one of your babies could swallow one. You have to think about things like that with twins; they can perform feats a single baby wouldn't dream of. Even when they were tiny infants, I'd watch as Kris twisted little decorations off of Johnny's outfit. If the boys had been unobserved, it could have been a problem, with one baby swallowing a tiny pompon or button.

For cooler weather, I liked long-sleeved T-shirts that snap in the front and come only to the tummy, to wear under other outfits. I wouldn't use the one-piece shirts under other clothing if I were you. If a diaper leaks, you have to change a whole outfit, and with two babies, you don't need any more outfit changes than necessary!

For newborns and older babies, stretchy one-piece pajamas are a godsend. I used them more often as play suits than as pajamas. Again, I loved having them in soft cotton, but I found that there were some very nice polyester blends available. The same goes for the little nightgowns with a drawstring at the bottom. That's what I swore by for sleeping when the boys were still newborns. They're great for changing a sleeping baby's diaper without waking him, especially if there's also a monitor attached to him. Just untie the string, slip the nightgown up, make the change and gently slide the gown down again. The drawstring closes the whole thing like a little bag, keeping the baby's feet warm, which I believe makes them sleep better.

Sleepwear Alert

When you're purchasing sleepwear for your babies be sure to look for pajamas or nightgowns that are flame resistant, which means that in the case of a fire, the garment will stop burning when removed from the fire itself. To conform with federal standards, cotton garments must be treated with a fire-resistant chemical; polyester fabrics must themselves be flame-resistant.

And speaking of those tiny feet, keep them warm all day with sock-type booties that pull on. They're not expensive—you can usually pick them up in the baby supply section at the grocery store. We color-coded the boys' booties for a while for simplicity's sake—one had all blue socks and one had all yellow socks. Kris and Johnny aren't identical, but I imagine that kind of color-coding could work for identical twins, for outfits as well as for booties—so long as everyone knows the code! For us, fewer colors meant that I could almost always put together a pair of socks, no matter how many the boys had managed to kick off and lose. I did find that those socks stayed on pretty well most of the time, and were much easier to deal with than booties that tie. Later, when they were learning to crawl and then to walk, and trying for traction on a slippery kitchen floor, I found similar sock-type booties with non-slip bottoms. The boys wore those indoors until they walked and switched to real shoes.

When your babies are newborns, you'll need lots of receiving blankets, which are just simple squares of soft flannel big enough to wrap a baby in. Here's one baby item that I think it's impossible to have too many of. While you're still in the hospital, you'll most likely learn about swaddling from the nurses. Most babies love to be swaddled, which means that they like to be wrapped up snug and tight in a receiving blanket. I suppose it's because they've just come out of the womb where snug and tight meant security—especially for twins. For whatever reason, most newborns don't seem to like to have their arms and legs freely flailing around, and receiving blankets offer the perfect way to make them feel cozy and safe.

In a few weeks, when your babies have outgrown the need to be swaddled, receiving blankets make a nice light stroller blanket or cover when they are sleeping. I also used them on the floor when the boys were old enough to be put down with a couple of toys for a little playtime.

By contrast, I had just one crib quilt per baby, and I felt that crib quilts were more for decoration than for really warming the baby. Besides, I always worried that one of the boys would wiggle around until his face was covered by the heavier quilt, and not be able to free himself, so I never used the quilts over the babies when they were sleeping. They really were redundant. When the weather was cool and the boys were past the newborn stage when they wore nightgowns, I'd dress them for bed in stretchy pajamas with blanket sleepers over them. Blanket sleepers for infants are like bags with arms and a zipper up the front you slip the baby into. My boys always kicked off any blanket I put over them, and with the sleepers I knew they were warm. Also, we had apnea monitors on them until they were five months old, and blankets just made it that much more difficult to keep the monitor on.

Another favorite item of mine for little babies was those flannel-covered waterproof pads. I had them in every size, from lap size to crib size. And I used them everywhere—on the couch if I was laying a baby down next to me, on my own lap, in the stroller and in their crib. Those pads saved lots of upholstery and dry cleaning bills for me, and I highly recommend them!

Don't you love the little warm hats they put on newborns to help them maintain their body temperature? I think tiny woolly hats are absolutely adorable, and even though I didn't get many for gifts, I was happy to go out and pick up several for the boys myself. They wore them all the time, indoors and out, for the first few weeks. I believe in hats for summer too. That tender baby skin needs all the protection you can give it, and my pediatrician said sunscreen is a no-no for very young babies. They'll suck it off their hands anyway and some ingredients, such as PABA may irritate their skin. So my boys always spent outdoor time in the shade, and they always wore hats, which I thought were so cute anyway.

Kris and Johnny never needed to wear snowsuits regularly because we live in California. But we have taken the boys to cold places on holiday, even when they were very small babies, and I can attest that snowsuits are truly a pain to get them into and out of, so think of how you'll do that before you buy one. One idea a friend shared that I find does help is that newborns don't really need to have their little arms threaded into the sleeves of snowsuits. Most babies are happier with their arms curled up close to their bodies anyway, and it's one less step involved in getting your babies ready to go out.

If you live in a cold climate, and your babies are born in the winter, you might try using a bunting, a cozy warm bag with arms (which you don't have to use) and a hood, for your babies while they are newborns. They are far easier than snowsuits to get babies into and out of. But look for buntings that have a special opening in the center for car seat straps, or you'll have a hassle trying to strap them in with all that extra fabric.

It makes me tired just to think of all that dressing and undressing we did with the boys. I can tell you I was extremely grateful we live in a warm climate. It means there's so much less clothing to squeeze them into. As long as I kept them safe from too much sun, life in that regard was pretty easy.

As you can see, there is plenty in the clothing and bedding department you will need for two babies. In addition to all of this, we were given dozens of hand-knitted outfits, which were all beautiful, thoughtful gifts. I'm a knitter myself, so I know how much skill these pieces required. I took photographs of the boys wearing their gifts, and made sure that everyone who sent us one received a picture. As a matter of fact, I discovered that's an easy way to send a thank you note that serves two purposes at once. Everyone wants pictures of your babies. If you add a few lines of thanks on the back of the photo, it can serve as a thank-you note. I'll be saving these knitted works of art to show to the boys when they're grown; they seemed almost too pretty to wear. Having a few special pieces of clothing that also carry sentimental value for your babies is wonderful. But remember: where the day-to-day is concerned, simplifying your twins' wardrobes will simplify your life.

What If I'm on Bed Rest and Can't Shop for My Babies?

If you have access to a computer, get on the Internet and order directly from companies who have web sites.

If you don't have a computer, have a friend collect catalogues which offer baby items, and settle in comfortably with the books and the phone. Or call all your favorite stores and reserve everything from furniture to clothing and arrange to buy them only after you or your husband has been able to see the items, or after the babies have been born.

For items you feel comfortable buying beforehand, pay with a credit card and have them delivered. Many stores as well as reputable catalogues have return policies that will allow you to return or exchange items that aren't right for you.

Fitting It All into the Nursery

Most of us, myself included, don't have a huge room set aside for the babies. So when we begin to see how much gear we're going to need for two babies, we realize it's going to be a bit of a trick to get in all in that room we've designated as the nursery.

Casey Kasem's wife, Jeannie, has a line of cribs she designs and sells. Their gift to us was two really beautiful round cribs. Some people feel that round cribs have an extra degree of safety because there are no corners for the baby to scoot into. We loved the round cribs, both the looks and the safety idea, but they took up a lot of space. They just didn't fit in the babies' room, so those went into the trailer on the set where they were used every single day, once I went back to work.

When we first brought Kris and Johnny home, they slept in little rocking bassinets instead of cribs. However, I have to say if you're on a budget, bassinets are probably a waste of money. The babies will be in them only for a matter of weeks, and then they'll grow right out of them. On the other hand, the bassinets did make it easy to transport the boys from room to room, or to have them in the room with me even if they were just sleeping, so they were useful for a short time. However there are ways to do the same thing, less expensively. Friends of mine transported their babies around the house in baby baskets, woven baskets with handles that are also called Moses Baskets. They could place the baskets on the floor near them, or on a sturdy table. If you really like the idea of cradles or bassinets for your babies, I'd suggest you borrow them if you can. Whether you buy them or borrow, be aware that sheets are a bit of an issue. I found that not all bassinets or cradles are standard sized, so you have to measure your mattress before you buy sheets.

You will need two cribs, although you might have your twins sleep together for a while when they are very small. Both of our boys slept in one crib at first. I liked the idea of them being together, and I think it was good for them. But after a couple of months, we put them in separate cribs. They'd just grown too big, and I was worried about the monitor wires getting tangled or coming loose.

Some people spend lots of money on fancy cribs, but to be honest, we did not. Ours were of good quality, but they were pretty basic. I spent more time, energy and money on having their room painted and choosing great fabric for the draperies and for the other furniture in the room than I did on buying and decorating the cribs. But everyone has their own way, and there are some beautiful cribs to choose from.

Can't I Just Borrow a Couple of Cribs or Get Them at a Tag Sale?

You can save money by borrowing cribs, but if you do, you must be aware of some safety issues. Be certain that the bars are no farther apart than 2⅜ inches. If the crib was made before 1978, there's probably a higher level of lead in the crib's original paint than is allowed today, and babies do chew on crib rails. Buy a new mattress and be sure the space between mattress and crib does not allow two adult fingers. Don't use a crib with cutouts in the headboard where a baby's hands or head can get caught. And don't use a crib with tall end posts on which a baby's clothing can get caught.

Since my first two children were born, stretchy cotton crib sheets have been developed that definitely help make it easier to change the sheets. I've even seen sheets with velcro ties instead of fitted corners. I always used one of those crib-sized waterproof felt pads under the sheet, and I'd put another under the babies' bottoms on top of the sheet to save changing the crib sheet every time one of them spit up or a diaper leaked.

You don't need pillows for your babies; it's too easy for babies to bury their faces in pillows and have trouble breathing. I used a soft clean cloth diaper under their heads. It kept the sheet from getting dirty every time they spit up.

Make a Wish List of What You Need

Make a master list of everything you think you'll need for your babies. Use it when you register for baby gifts at stores offering that service. Then cross off items when you have a baby shower or receive gifts in the mail. That way you'll have a running total of what you have and what you have left to collect. If friends ask what you need, you'll easily be able to give them a few suggestions.

On the same master list, you can make note of what you'll borrow and who you have borrowed an item from. Even though you think you'll never forget, in the whirl of activity and fatigue after your babies are born, it will be easier than you think to draw a blank when it's time to return the item.

We had the cribs delivered, which meant they came unassembled. I also had the delivery people assemble them, and I thought that service was definitely worth the extra charge. Cribs are not easy to put together, and if you do it yourself, you don't want to make a mistake and find the whole thing comes crashing down when you put a baby in it! Once the cribs were assembled, which we had them do right in the nursery, we saw that we had just enough room to put them end to end along one wall, with a changing table in between. That left us two walls for other furniture—the remaining wall having been taken up with doorways into the room and into the closet and bathroom. Along the longer of the two available walls, we placed a single bed with pillows arranged like a couch, which, if you have room is a wonderful addition to a nursery. It was perfect for lying down with one or two babies to nurse or just to nap. If you don't have that much room, I'd suggest you try to squeeze an easy chair in for nursing now, and for reading to them later.

You only need one rocking chair, and if it doesn't fit in the babies' room, I hope you can place it not too far away. And make sure your rocker is padded. You may be spending quite a bit of time in it, and it should be completely comfortable for you. I liked having a rocker with arms to support my arms, if I was nursing both boys at once.

The cribs, rocking chair, changing table and couch took up all the space in our nursery, so we put a dresser and shelves inside the boys' closet. There's just one small set of sturdy shelves in their room for books and toys.

The next most important purchase for the babies' room, after the cribs and rocking chair, is the changing table. A good sturdy one, with a changing platform at the right height for you will really save your back. Some people like the style that has open shelves below and a table on top. I like the kind that had dresser drawers below with a large fold-out surface on top. We never folded it in, and it was large enough to hold both babies at once, and had the added security of safety straps to hold one baby while we changed the other. When the boys grew bigger, we changed one at a time, but there was always plenty of room.

When it came to diapering, we used disposables. It was part of my "The simpler the better" philosophy. There just was so much work with two, we thought this was one way to make it a little easier. I know many people swear by diaper services, which bring clean cloth diapers to your door. But for me it just seemed like *so* many diapers to deal with, so we went with the disposables.

However, we did find lots of other uses for those cloth diapers. The most important one was as a security object for the boys. When they were tiny, still in the hospital I think, I started giving each a clean, soft cloth diaper to cuddle up with. I know that doesn't sound very interesting, but I think it was just the best thing and the boys seemed fine with it. Cloth diapers are, after all, interchangeable and if one became soiled I could easily toss it in the laundry, in the meantime substituting a clean "security object" for the dirty one. I liked this approach especially when they were newborn, and I was particularly careful about things being absolutely clean for them. The beauty of it was you could always find a "blankie," and it would be clean. I've seen other parents go through enormous trauma when The Stuffed Rabbit or The Shredded Blanket was missing, or so filthy they were worried about it. Our boys had the cloth diapers, and they worked well.

We also used rolled up cloth diapers for propping the boys in their beds so they could lie on their sides when they were newborns. Some parents use a special wedge-shaped pillow for propping, but I thought the diapers worked just fine.

Last, but definitely not least, one of the best things I did in decorating the nursery was to have a dimmer switch installed. Dim light allowed me to check on the babies without waking them, change a diaper without glaring lights, or even to calm the mood a bit as we got them ready for bed. A small lamp would work too, but the dimmer just seemed the height of convenience to me.

Bathing Your Babies

James and I have loved to bathe Kris and Johnny since the first day we were able to, when their umbilical cords fell off. From that day forward, bathing them has been more than just another chore we must do. When they were too tiny to bathe them together, I would bathe Johnny while James held Kris, and then we'd switch. I loved just about everything about bathing them, from holding them securely in the water where you could see their tight little fists loosen and open, like tiny flowers blooming; to wrapping them in those little hooded towels afterwards. And the scent of a newly washed baby must be the closest thing to heaven we can experience here on earth.

James and I still do the evening bath whenever we can. If we have been gone a lot, traveling or working, or if the day has simply been rocky, bath time is our time together, our time to smooth everything out. It's also part of a larger ritual that ends with tucking a comforter cozily around each squirming boy, and wishing him well on his trip to dreamland. Of course in our house, with boys who are now four years old, the ritual doesn't always end that peacefully! But whatever the ending, bath time provides a calm beginning and a chance for us to quite literally reconnect, physically and emotionally, with the boys.

When they first came home from the hospital, we bathed them in a plastic tub we set on the sink counter in the bathroom off their bedroom. I liked to use one of those baby-sized sponges in the bottom of the plastic tub. It seemed to me that the sponge kept the baby warm because he lay directly upon it, and it conformed a little bit to the shape of his body. But even if I only imagined that, I know the sponge made it less likely that I would drop him. Babies in bathtubs are very slippery little creatures, and even a quick slither from your hands to a hard plastic tub surface can frighten or hurt the baby.

I've never been one to use a lot of scented creams or washes on my babies' skin. For the most part they just don't need it, and you never know if a cream will actually irritate that tender new skin. We did have a lot of diaper rashes when the boys were very small, and the one exception I made to adding things to their bath was powdered vitamin C. You can buy it at any health food store, and I found that its antioxidant properties helped heal rashes. I'd just sprinkle it in the water when they bathed, and then of course use some kind of a barrier cream with zinc oxide in it before I diapered them.

If you can believe it, even with all the redecorating we did to convert the boys' bedroom from a guest room to a nursery, we'd really not thought until the last minute about the fact that their bathroom held only a shower. So we quickly had it taken out and a bathtub put in. Because we did it that way, we had the luxury of adding a few features we knew from experience would make it easier to bathe the boys as babies, toddlers and older. First, we made sure the tub itself would be large enough for two children.

Although we bathed them separately as infants, I always imagined they'd be bathing together later—much more time efficient for us and more fun for them. Then, we had the tub lined with a non-skid mosaic tile so it wouldn't be slippery, and we made sure there was enough deck space all around the tub for storing their toys. That plan worked almost too well. If you were to peek into the boys' bathroom this evening, you'd see that there are so many toys in the tub with them, they can barely move! It's a little ridiculous I'll admit, but the prospect of being immersed in toys as well as water makes them happily trot off to the bath whenever we say it's time.

Johnny and Kris have always loved having baths as much as we love giving them. All my children have. Perhaps it's because they've enjoyed being in their baths so much that they've never been afraid of having water in their faces. I did make a point of letting small amounts of water splash on their faces when they were very young, so water in the face was never a big issue. Later, when it came to dealing with much more water such as swimming underwater, or washing their hair, it was an easy transition.

Another great part about bathing the babies has been that Sean and Katie have taken part, creating one more fun way for them to connect with the boys. Ever since Johnny and Kris were quite small, their brother and sister either helped with bathing, or put on their bathing suits and hopped right in with the boys! It can be a real three-ring circus with all of them splashing around in the much larger tub in the master bathroom.

Getting Around

Getting out with two babies, particularly if you are alone, can be a real challenge. Mercifully, there is quite a broad selection of helpful equipment available. Still, I'd recommend that you try before you buy any item if it's at all possible. While some types of equipment can be quite expensive, still, certain things are truly essential when you're taking care of two. Once you've decided an item is going to be indispensable for you, place it at the very top of the wish list you let your family and friends know about.

I'd say that the single most useful piece of baby equipment I've ever used—with each of my babies, not just with twins—was the Snugli baby carrier. I was given one as a gift when Katie was born, and I have used one with each of my babies since then. For the uninitiated, a Snugli is a pouch in which you can comfortably carry your baby on the front of your body, supported by a belt that ties around your waist, and broad straps that cross over your shoulders in the back. Some models allow you to switch the baby to your back when he gets beyond the newborn stage.

Because we were experienced Snugli users, when the boys came we bought two of them and simply strapped them on together to "wear" both babies at once. I wore them for a while, but my nanny most often wore them once I went back to work, while the babies were still small. Snuggled cozily into their own little cloth pouch, the boys definitely were happy campers. The whole arrangement worked brilliantly, even with the monitors. For calming fussy babies at home, we found we could rock them, wearing both in the Snugli, with the wires that led to the monitors arranged over our shoulders.

Later when I was back on the set of *Dr. Quinn,* there was one episode in which Michaela's baby was given a lovely leather sling by the Indians. I couldn't resist trying it out with one of my own boys, and it worked beautifully. I can't quite imagine wearing two slings in order to carry twins, but the arrangement made me think about the fabric slings that are available now. They seem to be quite comfortable and might be worth a try, especially if you can handle carrying one baby that way and pushing the other in a stroller.

On the show, Michaela's baby had a gorgeous wicker pram, which of course we tried out on the boys as well, wheeling them around the set between takes. We even dressed them in period costumes and photographed them in the pram. It was very sweet, but nothing could compare with the side-by-side jogging stroller we had for the boys. We desperately needed something far more rugged than a delicate pram, or even than a regular stroller. After all, the set for *Dr. Quinn* was located in a state park, and that's where we took the babies every work day. We needed something rugged enough to go

Stroller or Carriage—How Do I Decide?

Choosing the right type of baby transportation for your needs is so important when you have twins. It can make the difference between feeling house-bound and cabin-fevered during the first year or two of their lives, and feeling that you can actually rejoin the world with your babies in tow.

Here are some things to think about as you choose:

- A carriage is like a bed on wheels—comfy but bulky and not easily folded to fit into a car trunk, or to lug up bus steps. If you have one from a previous baby, two infants will probably fit in it for a while.
- Strollers come in several styles for twins. In-line strollers have two seats (or three if you have another young child) which face each other or all face front. Side-by-side strollers also come in two or three seats, but can be difficult to maneuver through doorways. In either case, it's wise to get one with seats that recline for very young babies, and sit up for when they get older.
- Try your choice out in the store before you buy it. Can you steer it with one hand? Can you fold it up easily? When it's folded, can you carry it easily? Does it have brakes you can rely on to hold the stroller or carriage in place? Does it seem sturdy and stable, not easy to tip over? Is the handle adjustable so that it can be set to the right height for you and for your husband or baby-sitter? Does it have a place where you can stash purchases or the diaper bag? How about a rain/wind shield?

on trails, over rocks and boulders without having to worry about the wheels falling off or the babies falling out. In fact, with its big wheels we could run with that stroller, jog with it, or climb mountains with it. We also needed a stroller that allowed us to cover the boys completely to shade them from the sun and wind, and this one had a canopy and rain shield that did just that.

One of my favorite photos of the boys and me involves that stroller. It was taken when the boys were about six weeks old. We were doing a photo shoot for *McCall's* magazine, and searching for a fresh way to show a mother and her new babies. Kris and Johnny were still so tiny, and we hit on the idea of putting them in their big red jogging stroller, which of course dwarfed them at that age. Weeks before the shoot, the stylist brought me the dress I was to wear—this slim, red satin Chinese gown which you wouldn't wear unless you were in great shape—it shows everything. I would have chosen something else but the stylist loved it, and it happened to match the stroller perfectly. My consolation was that I had a few weeks to work at getting back in shape before they did the shoot. The photo turned out very elegant and very tongue in cheek at the same time. We shot it in the garage at my house, of all places, looking very cool and glamorous in that red gown, holding a bottle for one of the babies.

Jane's Top Ten List of Baby Gear Essentials

Most of these are things I've used, that have made my life with twins so much easier. A few are items I've seen friends use, and if I had it to do over again, I'd use them myself.

10. **One quiet rocking chair**—comfortably padded, with no squeaks to wake sleeping babies.
 9. **Two bouncy baby chairs**—because babies love to bounce in these chairs made of strong wire frames supporting a fabric hammock. I've seen babies bounce happily while their

parents manage to eat their entire dinner, undisturbed.

8. **One baby swing**—if you can't fit two in your living room—and how many people can—one will let you deal with your babies singly once in a while.

7. **One jumper toy**—hanging from the molding over a doorway, this crazy toy can keep older babies (five months and up) happy for ages. But you can't leave your baby untended, which is actually fine. We loved watching our jumping boys!

6. **One set of nursery monitors**—so that you can hear them even if you're outdoors. If your home is small, it's not a necessity. But if they're upstairs and you're downstairs, it's a godsend.

5. **One or two baby carriers**—but try out a double model before you buy it. All but the tiniest babies may be too heavy for you to carry comfortably. A single baby pouch and a single stroller may be a better combination.

4. **One easy-to-use and transport** baby stroller.

3. **One breast pump**—the highest quality you can afford to buy, rent, or borrow. I rented mine.

2. **Someone to do the laundry**—a friend who comes over to do your laundry a couple of times a week for a month is the best shower gift I've ever heard of.

And the most vital item to have when you're given the great gift of twins:

1. **One truly wonderful, helpful husband!**

eight

Stepping into the World

After months of carrying your twins safely inside your body, and then a couple more months at home with them, it may seem difficult to let your little ones out into the world. Even if that means going only as far as your day care provider or to a friend's house for a play date. After all, *out there* is full of unpredictable people and as many dangers as your heart and mind can conjure, to say nothing of germs!

But that *is* our main responsibility with children, isn't it: To give them a loving, secure start and then to help them find their place in the larger world, one baby step at a time. For the most part, it's a delightful task, full of wonder and surprise for an observant parent. But there is that darker side, a certain type of worry that mothers always seem to have about the welfare of their children. I found that by setting up an environment for my boys that I believed was nurturing and right for them, I could put my mind at ease—even if I wasn't with them.

In the months after your babies are born, I know you'll be thinking about what comes next, for them and for you. Don't be surprised if how you feel now is completely different from how you thought you would feel, particularly if these are your first babies. Once you have held your babies in your arms, I wouldn't be surprised if you were ready to reevaluate your plans to return to work as quickly as you thought you would. I've known women who have, with their spouses, reworked the family budget so they could stay home with their babies for a while. On the other hand, I've known those who planned to stay home who felt the changes just as strongly, and who found that they needed more help than they'd predicted, or that they longed for more adult contact than they thought they would. And I've known those who gave up work entirely to be home with their babies.

The point is that I believe no one can really foresee how she will feel when she becomes a mother. Although I was already a mother when my twins were born, I found that the impact of two babies on my life was more enormous than I'd thought it would be. Having two babies was really *more* of everything—I was *more* tired, *more* stressed, *more* overwhelmed than I'd been with one baby. I hope that after your babies are born, you'll allow yourself the time and the open-mindedness to revisit whatever plans you'd made for stepping back into your world, in order to see clearly what will be the right situation for you and for your babies.

Life with Babies

Your life with babies for the first couple of months should be one of learning their rhythms, and doing all you can to aid in your own recovery from the pregnancy and birth. When I had each of my single born children, it seemed I didn't need to be particularly mindful of my health and energy after the baby came. Of course I was younger then, but still, recovery just seemed to happen.

With Johnny and Kris I focused much more clearly on my health and theirs during their first two months. Even if you do not have the complications I did, when you have twins I think it's a good idea to keep those first months as calm and focused as possible. You do have the habits of two babies to learn, and if your twins are fraternal, they are likely to have very different habits indeed. Identical twins may also behave very differently, even at this early age, but they are more likely to have similar bio-rhythms—getting hungry at the same time, nursing for similar amounts of time, and even sleeping in tandem. In any case, I found it does take some patience and care to observe all this about your babies, and really get to know both of them during these months. Minimizing outside responsibilities will help you to do that. And, if it's possible for you to stretch your maternity leave so that you can stay home a bit longer, that would be good too.

My maternity leave lasted a little more than two months, which was great. In reality I had little choice about returning to work, or even about delaying my return to work because I was under contract, and a shooting schedule involving a couple hundred people had already been set. But that was compensated for by the fact that I had one of the best child care situations one could possibly dream of. When I returned to work, with the help of a nanny I was easily able to have Johnny and Kris with me at the set every day.

The baby trailer on the *Dr. Quinn* set was a perfectly clean baby-safe environment, so while I was out in the dust and dirt with the horses, I didn't worry for a minute about my tiny infants, because I knew they were safely sheltered. Between rehearsals and takes, I spent every spare moment back at the trailer, washing up and then playing with them, changing them, and feeding them. I still had plenty of work to do on the set, but at least I could spend time sitting in a quiet, air conditioned trailer with a nursing baby in one arm, while I held a script in my other hand, learning lines for the next scene. Because of the apnea monitors they wore for five months, the boys spent much of their early months inside the trailer, but we could also take them out in the sturdy double jogging stroller. The stroller was large enough, and the babies were small enough that we could fit the monitors in with them and take them around for walks and fresh air.

When the boys no longer needed the monitors, they began to have a more typical babyhood, and then toddler life. Actually *typ-*

ical is probably not the right word, now that I think of it. They were typical children, but the lives they had were anything *but* typical. Because they were with me on the set, the pretend world millions of people saw portrayed each week on *Dr. Quinn, Medicine Woman* became their real world. There in a beautiful, safe state park, we had created the atmosphere of a particularly gentle 19th century frontier town, with the important addition of 20th century comforts. In many ways, the set was just like a small town of a hundred years ago. Everyone knew everyone else, and we all truly cared about one another. There was always someone who wanted to play with Johnny and Kris, so they were never bored, always engaged.

By the time the boys were three or four months old, we could unhook the monitors for a few moments, and we were sitting them on horses, where they could ride around propped in front of a wrangler or someone we knew would be careful with them. Or we'd pull them around in one of the old-fashioned wagons we used on the show. Luke, Lesa's boy, became their best friend, and we'd have all three children together in the wagon so we could move them from place to place on the set. And of course the triplet girls who played Michaela Quinn's child were on the set every day too, so the three boys and the three girls played together all the time.

Whenever we weren't filming in a large open area of the set called the big meadow, the children were out there in the meadow running around, playing. By the time my boys were a little more than a year old, it seems there had been a baby boom among cast and crew. So many people, including Beth Sullivan with her twins, had new babies; I think the final tally was nine little ones. Lunch time at the meadow looked like a preschool at recess! The children were so adorable we decided to use all of them in one episode. It was the one in which Michaela Quinn and Sully are celebrating their child's first birthday with a picnic. We had all the children, and Beth too, dressed up in period costume. Nineteenth century boys were dressed in clothing that looks very feminine to our eyes, so it was particularly amusing to see our rough-and-tumble little boys toddling around in frills and lace. It was a lovely, memorable day—bright quilts spread on the grass, toddlers squealing and running everywhere, their fingers sticky with birthday cake icing. What an amazing mix of 19th and 20th century fun!

When the boys were nearly two years old, they started going down to the creek with their nanny to throw stones in the water, or to play pirates and shipwrecks, or to go fishing. Oh, they had lots of adventures out there. To this day, whenever they watch a *Dr. Quinn* episode on video, they get very excited because to them, they're not just watching a television show, they're seeing their favorite play area.

Your Postpartum Body

Let me assure you that as unfamiliar as your life may be for you after your twins are born, your body is likely to feel even stranger. If you've done as your doctor no doubt asked in your pregnancy, you've gained quite a bit of weight. Of course we hope every one of those calories goes directly to the babies, but honestly, that's not always the case. Most new twin moms I know are quite distressed when they get on the scale a week or so after the birth. For most of us, the weight of two babies may be gone, as well as that of their placentas, but that's about it. Losing 20 pounds or so in a couple of weeks may sound wonderful to mothers of one baby, but in the face of a 40 or 50 pound weight gain, a 20-pound loss seems not nearly so significant.

Unlike most mothers of twins, my baby weight did disappear rather quickly, but it wasn't because of any effort I made to lose weight. I had barely gained enough weight for twins in the first place, not for lack of trying. Dr. Ross would have liked me to gain about 10 or 15 pounds more than I did, but despite my best efforts, I just could not. After the birth I was still so ill, and then there were difficulties getting my digestive system to work correctly again, so the quick weight loss wasn't surprising.

I can't offer you an overnight solution to dropping your baby weight, and I don't recommend the way I lost it! But I can assure

How Soon Will I Feel Like My Old Self After the Babies Come?

Think of it this way: It took nine months (or a little less) for your body to change so dramatically while you were pregnant. It is likely to take at least nine months to reverse those changes. During that time, your hormones will slowly be returning to pre-pregnant levels, so you may experience wide emotional swings: euphoric one moment, numb and exhausted the next, overwhelmed and worried right after that.

Your body needs time to recover in other ways too. For example, it will take at least six weeks for your uterus to shrink back to its pre-pregnant size. If you gained fifty pounds or more, you may lose about twenty of it in the first few weeks. It should take three to four months or longer to lose the other thirty. If you are nursing, your breasts are likely to remain larger and your body is likely to hold on to that last 10 pounds until you stop.

Try to think of the post-pregnancy process not only in terms of losing weight, but also in terms of regaining a basic level of tone and muscle to support your posture and mobility. You may have lost more muscle than you think during your pregnancy through inactivity or through the extreme stretching your abdominal muscles had to do to accommodate two babies.

you that with healthy eating (not overeating), in time it will go. I like to eat plenty of protein, and lots of fruits and vegetables, as a basis for a healthy life. If you're nursing, please don't try to lose weight until your babies are weaned; it will only damage your health. If you're not nursing, you should still eat in a healthful way so you'll have the energy to take care of those babies. Patience and time are key in facing post-baby weight. And the right kinds of exercise will help too.

Even though working out is not my favorite thing to do, I'm a believer in appropriate exercise, both for regaining strength and tone, and for regaining energy. Brigitta Gallo, my personal trainer during my pregnancy, came to the hospital three days after the boys were born to talk to me about exercising.

"You must be crazy!" I remember saying when she said it was time to start working out again.

But, she wasn't crazy at all, and the appropriate workout turned out to be rather subtle isometric exercises that came with Dr. Ross' blessing. That day, she had me doing Kegels and two other isometric exercises. I had been doing Kegels quite frequently just before the birth, so it wasn't too difficult to pick them up again. The fact that I'd had a cesarean helped, because those muscles hadn't been involved in the birth. After a vaginal birth, I remember that even locating those muscles afterward took a great deal of focus.

Birgitta also gave me an isometric for my abdominals, in which I would simply lie on my back with my knees bent and feet on the floor, pull in my abdominal muscles and hold them to a count of 10 or 15, or longer if I could. Because they had been so stretched by the pregnancy, this simple move was difficult at first—it really required some concentration.

The third isometric was a pelvic tilt, which I could also do lying on my back, again with both knees bent and my feet on the floor. Birgitta had me pull in my abs, squeeze my glutes, and curve my lower back to tilt my pelvis upward. I'd do this ten times, twice a day. They may not sound like much, but these isometrics were effective and they really set my muscles on the road to recovery.

Still, I was left with a pouchy little tummy, which I carried the whole time I was breast feeding. It's basically gone now, although if I sit down and slouch forward, you can see that where the babies were, the skin is crepey. When I look down at my own abdomen now, I marvel at the fact that these two husky four-year-olds once grew there. I can't imagine where all that skin went! Some women do have quite a bit of loose tummy skin left after they have twins, and I suppose one could have cosmetic surgery to have the excess skin removed. But I find that if I stand up straight, that bit of excess skin I have disappears, thank goodness. So my recommendation for minimizing post-twin-tummy-skin is to exercise, stand straight, and don't wear a bikini!

Getting back in shape quickly is a requirement in my business, and it was a good thing I started to do that in the safest way possible soon after the boys were born. I never know when something is going to come up that requires me to look glamorous, new babies or no. Sure enough, at 6:00 A.M., two weeks after the boys were born, the phone rang and I answered it, a little annoyed at such an early morning call. But my annoyance melted immediately when I heard someone on the other end of the line say, "Congratulations! You've been nominated for a Golden Globe Award!"

The last thing on my mind at that time was my career. I was not thinking whatsoever about work or awards; it was all babies and diapers and nursing for me. But once the idea took hold, I was thrilled that I had been nominated for *Dr. Quinn*. I remember thinking, "Isn't this exciting! *And* I just had twins. How many more wonderful things could happen?"

If anything could have dampened my spirits then, it was the fact that the ceremony was only five weeks away. Now that was a sobering thought. I already knew I needed to get in shape to be able to wear the slim red Chinese gown we'd planned to use for the *McCall's* shoot, so I decided that would also be my Golden Globes gown. One of my first phone calls after finding out I'd been nominated was to Birgitta, and we started immediately, working like crazy in my small home gym to get me back in shape. Here was a challenge with a couple of hugely important goals. I wanted not only to work out in the safest way possible considering I'd just had twins, but I also wanted to be able to stand confidently in a slinky red gown in front of millions of people, and not worry that my stomach was sticking out!

How Soon Can I Begin Exercising After a Cesarean Birth?

If you had a cesarean, your workout will be different than if you had your babies vaginally. Of course you must have your doctor's approval before you do any kind of exercise.

Several days after a cesarean birth you can do:

- **Kegels** to strengthen the muscles of your pelvic floor which supported the weight of two babies for all those months.
- **Pelvic tilts** to relieve tightness in the lower back and to help strengthen your abdominal muscles as well as your buttocks. Lie on your back with both knees bent and your feet on the floor. Squeeze your abs and glutes, curve your pelvis upward, rounding the lower back. Do this 10 times, twice a day.

A week after a cesarean birth you can add:

- **Pelvic hip lifts** using the same form as a tilt, but lifting your hips off the floor.
- **Foot exercises** to promote circulation. Point, flex and circle your feet in all directions.

If you have your doctor's approval, you can start a regular exercise program after two to four weeks.

The other complication of trying to look great after having twins in general—and in the Chinese dress in particular—had to do with breast feeding. Not only were my breasts much larger than normal, but I had to figure out how to put breast pads into my bra so that they wouldn't show in this very slim gown, and so that I wouldn't leak at an inauspicious moment. Ironically, the last time I'd won a Golden Globe was right after Katie was born, and although I certainly was open to winning the award again, I very much hoped I didn't repeat the embarrassing performance I'd given then. I'd been completely stunned when my name was announced as the winner. When I was handed the award on live television, I burst into tears and said, "I want to thank my new baby Katie because I know she's missing me because my milk just came in . . ."

I've seen that clip of me crying and saying my milk just came in (it seems everyone plays it every chance they get) . . . and I have to say it is definitely embarrassing. So with my second nomination for a Golden Globe, I really didn't want to tell the world whether or not my milk was coming in—and I didn't want that milk making splotches on the front of my dress on national television.

After weeks of work with Birgitta, on the night of the Golden Globes James zipped me into that dress smooth as could be, and I deftly positioned the pads in my bra the way I'd practiced, so I wouldn't worry about leakage. I really felt the chances of my winning were zero because family shows like *Dr. Quinn* rarely get that kind of attention. But whether or not I won an award later that evening, I knew I looked the way I'd wanted to in that dress, and that was almost triumph enough. I consoled myself with the thought that no matter what happened that night, James and I would at least have a much-needed evening out. That's why, I suppose, that when they announced my name, I really couldn't believe it. I didn't move from my seat until James looked at me and said, "You won!" I was beside myself with excitement. But this time I had the presence of mind to make a more traditional acceptance speech, and I said not a word about my milk, although I did mention Kris and Johnny.

Jane's Postpartum Workout

In order to be safe about postpartum workouts, think of yourself as still pregnant for the first two to three months after the birth. Hormones left from pregnancy will still be making your joints loose, so your balance and coordination may be off. Check with your doctor before you begin any kind of workout after having your babies.

Jane worked on her abdominal muscles in a variety of ways, beginning with **isometric abdominal contractions** and **pelvic tilts.** A week later, she added **abdominal curls,** which are the same as the pelvic tilt with the addition of lifting or curling the shoulders and head off the floor to about 30 degrees, arms extended forward or behind your head.

After a week of those exercises, Jane was able to resume the pregnancy workout described in Chapter 3, with continued emphasis on safety and working specifically on strengthening her abdominal muscles, buttocks and the muscles of her upper back, which were sore and tired from nursing.

Your Famous Babies

The most immediate result of that evening at the Golden Globes was that the entire world definitely knew I'd had twins. James said that anyone who didn't know about Johnny and Kris at that point must have been living under a rock!

While I'm well aware that my life with twins is different from what most people experience, one thing I believe we all share is the instant fame that twins bring to every family within their own circle of friends and relatives. We all lose our own identities a bit after we have twins, and for a while we become known not so much as ourselves any more, but as Parents of Twins. Wherever I go now people say, "How are the twins?" It used to be, "Oh I saw you in that movie!" or "I love *Dr. Quinn,*" or maybe, "Aren't you Jane Seymour?" Not any more. The same has happened to my father-in-law. He is the well-known actor and television personality Stacy Keach Sr., a wonderful man who has had a long and well-respected acting career. Now he does so many television commercials his face and voice are instantly recognizable to millions of people. But since the boys were born, all of that takes second place.

"Once, I had my own identity," he loves to tell me with a twinkle in his eye, "but now that's all gone. I'm the grandfather to the twins now."

All of this goes to show how much these little guys have taken over all our lives. In doing so, it's clear to me how much they have the ability to bring us all down to earth, no matter what our professions are, or what our lives were like before they were born. To James and I, the attention the boys get is a gentle reminder of what a great gift they are to us and to our family.

I think most adults take that in stride. At least that's the way it happened in our house. As a mom or dad or grandparent, you are so proud of those babies, it doesn't hurt a bit to have everyone else acknowledge how wonderful they are. But I really was concerned about my other children. The changes for them in the two years before the boys were born had been enormous. Not only did Katie and Sean now have a new stepdad, James, living with us, but now they also had to deal with these famous babies. Both James and I did our best during the pregnancy and right after the boys were born to involve Katie and Sean in the pregnancy and in their care, and to continually reassure them in every way we could that they wouldn't lose their places of importance for us. That all seemed to be working out. But after we brought the babies home we seemed to be entering another era, and I was very watchful to see how Katie and Sean reacted as the newness wore off and the babies simply became their little brothers.

I'm happy to say that the early reassurance for Katie and Sean must have had a good effect. Both of them became so positively obsessed with Johnny and Kris, so excited and proud of them, they could barely keep their hands off the boys. They wanted to take the babies to school for show and tell—the babies might as well have been puppies! Friends simply had to come over to see them, to hold them, to play with them, even to change them.

For Sean, it was especially important that his biological dad would love those babies. And David did fall in love with them. Sean told me David had said soon after meeting the babies, "I don't know what it is, but those twins are the cutest things I've ever seen!" Babies do seem to have a way of really bringing people together and David's love for Kris and Johnny definitely strengthened his relationship with all of us. We'd all go together to Sean's baseball games, and once David had gotten to know the babies, he'd automatically grab one of them to hold on his lap as if he were the dad. I suppose it might have looked a little strange to an outsider, but at Sean's games I would be sitting there with James on one side holding a baby and David on the other, holding the other baby!

I hope you're ready for the attention you'll get for having twins, and your babies will get for being twins. While it can be quite a nice reminder of how lucky we all are who have twins, unwanted attention can also at times be annoying. A friend of mine who is very shy told me that all the attention truly bothered her. She just did not like all the fuss or the fact that total strangers would come up and want to hold one of her babies, or delay her as she was trying to get her errands done. She took to bringing just one baby at a time with her when she went out, although that didn't always work because it meant she had to have someone care for the other one. It seemed silly to bring a baby on a quick errand to the bank when there was a babysitter at home with the other one! Finally she decided on using a single stroller for one baby and carrying the other in a front pouch or a backpack. She found that fewer people noticed they were twins, and she could go about her business in peace.

Attention is one of the things that everyone in my family is accustomed to. During the time right after the babies were born, we had so many requests for photo shoots and magazine interviews we could barely keep track of them. Thankfully, I had years before developed my own personal set of rules about how to handle those requests.

I worked this out after Katie was born. At first, I swore my children would never be photographed publicly. Then the day after she was born I was asked to pose with Katie for a tiny photograph to be used in *Time* magazine with a story about celebrities breast feeding their babies. It seemed like such a good cause to

---

Behind the Scenes with the Gerber Babies

When Kris and Johnny were just under a year old, Gerber asked if the three of us could do some commercials together. It was really quite a fun project, full of surprises. We shot the commercials on the *Dr. Quinn* set, because that's where we were all day anyway, and the boys were perfectly at home there.

At one point there was a rather long speech I had to give, looking into the camera while holding two squirming boys on my lap. To amuse the boys and keep their attention, someone on the crew played a Barney videotape so that it showed on the screen just above the camera where the prompter usually showed the script. So when Kris and Johnny looked at the camera, they saw Barney. Unfortunately so did I. And, there was no room for the words I had to say, so I had to remember the lines *and* try not to laugh at Barney.

---

promote, I waived my short-lived rule and agreed to do the shoot. "Just this once," I told myself.

Then, wouldn't you know, when Katie was about three months old, I got a call from *Vogue* and they too wanted to do a shoot with Katie and me. I remember thinking, "Well gosh, how am I going to tell my daughter when she's a teenager that I turned down *Vogue* for her?" So I agreed to do that shoot too. The funny thing was that I was expecting to wear beautiful gowns, but they had me wearing torn exercise gear most of the time! It was all done at Canyon Ranch spa, which was wonderful, and the pictures turned out to be some of my favorites; gorgeous studies of mother and child.

James was there too, and he is so brilliant in dealing with the boys. Kris was getting a little fussy, but luckily James had his harmonica in his pocket, because he plays. So he gave it to Kris to keep him happy until we finished the shoot. That's why, in that particular commercial, you can see Kris at the end, playing the harmonica.

During the same shoot, after the second or third take I heard this cheer, and applause from the crew after they'd played back a previous take. When I had time to watch it, I saw what they were cheering about. Just when I'd said, "Shouldn't your baby be a Gerber baby?" Johnny had looked at me and nodded yes. Then Kris looked at the camera and made one of his cute little faces, sort of a Gerber pout. We couldn't have coached them to behave more perfectly.

All of which goes to show that when you're working with children, a lot has to do with how lucky you happen to be that day!

From those early shoots with Katie, I did finally develop my own set of rules, which have served all of us well: Katie and Sean, and now Johnny and Kris. You too may find that you're asked to have your twins photographed someday. If you are, you'll want to give some thought to it before you agree, and perhaps my experience will be helpful in making your decision. Here's what I've done to be sure any work my children do isn't harmful to them:

- I always tell whoever is doing the shoot that if the babies aren't happy about it, if they cry or seem distressed, we abandon the shoot. That's my first rule—the child's comfort reigns.
- James and I pick and choose—we certainly don't do anywhere near all the requests I get for interviews and photos either for me or for the children.
- We maintain control over which photos are published by having one photographer we know and trust take a series of shots of us and of the boys in a nice location somewhere when we're on vacation. He then sells them to different magazines, so we are not constantly hounded for photos.

From the beginning, we have simply refused to run from one magazine to another or from one photographer to another. By using our own selection of photographers and keeping an up-to-date collection of photos available for magazines that want them, we have kept control over publicity we're bound to get anyway. The result has been that the magazines get what they want without sending photographers to jump out of bushes at us, although once in a while someone still surprises us. It seems we've reached a reasonable compromise: Rather than refusing to have any photos taken of my children, I simply control what gets taken and what gets used.

Looking Good, Feeling Good

I'd say those first weeks after you have twins have to be the most difficult time in a variety of ways. You are most likely extremely exhausted, and your old body is still a dim, pre-pregnancy memory.

This is a time to be particularly nice to yourself. If it's possible, don't even look at your maternity clothing—you're probably sick of all of it anyway, and it's depressing to think that most of it still fits. Instead, buy or borrow a few pieces of clothing in an in-between size to help you feel fresh and pretty again. You'll have to really reevaluate sizes and decide what will work for now, now that your breasts are big and belly isn't so big. Cheri made a couple of solid recommendations for me after the boys were born, and I find she has an unfailingly great sense of what will be flattering even under the most difficult of circumstances. She suggested I try wearing a straight shell, not fitted and not too long so it wouldn't emphasize larger hips, with a soft blouse over it to minimize what was left of that post-pregnancy belly and over-sized bust. It was easy to nurse in that, and I could wear it with tights or comfortable pants. I also wore some big sweaters with tights, but I felt more like I was getting back to my old self if I didn't wear really enormous or baggy things on top.

The larger issue during those early months after the boys were born was my hair. As an older mom, I was in the classic, good news/bad news situation. The good news was that while I was pregnant I had grown a ton of hair and it was thick and luxurious for months. The bad news was that once the boys were born, suddenly, I had a new crop of gray hairs!

I also lost quite a bit of hair after they were born, which is typical. Don't panic if that's what's happening to you; it's part of a normal process. Dr. Ross told me I grew that extra gorgeous hair during pregnancy because of hormones and increased blood volume. After the pregnancy, when everything else about my body was returning to normal, my hair did as well, which accounts for the fall-out. Please take comfort in knowing that eventually everything normalizes, including hair, and some of what you may have lost will grow back, as mine did. But as it does, it may seem to come back in tufts, however that's only because you'll be dealing with two lengths of hair at once: hair of your normal length and areas of the brand-new, half-inch-long hair.

If the new hair is very obvious, one solution is to cut all your hair shorter. I completely understand anyone cutting her hair when she is pregnant or when she has small children. I have one friend who confided that she cut her very long hair when her twins were infants. "I feel like I'm always looking down at them through a tunnel of hair," she explained. So perhaps you will feel that it's time for a change anyway, and a new shorter style will be just right for you. Still, I would caution against going too short while you're pregnant.

Besides, having suddenly short hair if you're used to long hair may be too drastic a change at this moment, when everything else in your life is changing so fast. I wanted to leave my hair long, so it became a question of how to style my hair so I could deal with these strange tufts. What did I do? I simply learned how to wear it up, or partially up during that time until the tufts grew long enough so the casual observer wouldn't notice there were bits sticking out.

I've always chosen to have long hair because I feel I have more possibility of variation with longer hair, and that really saved me when I was dealing with those tufts. I can tie it back and it disappears completely, or I can have it loose and long, or in various combinations of those things. But you want the *real* reason, the truth about why I don't cut my hair? It's very simple. I hate going to the hairdresser! I hate fixing my hair, and I think shorter hair is more work. There is usually a lot of styling and blowing dry to do with shorter hair, and you have to keep up with haircuts. I don't do any of that, except the occasional trim to get rid of dry ends. Most days I don't do anything to my hair but wash it, condition it and let it dry naturally. The one downside of my long hair is that my boys have been known to grab and pull, which I can attest is quite painful!

During this time of change and adjustment, I believe a little self-pampering is in order. At first when the boys were born, I thought it would be a struggle to keep up much of my previous beauty regime, and that it might be selfish or frivolous to try very hard to devote time like that to myself anyway. Soon though, I discovered I was wrong. I badly needed the peace and quiet, I needed the time alone, and I needed to feel that I was being taken care of too, even if it was I who was doing the caring. I decided to try a short at-home spa day for myself. After the very first one, I definitely felt rejuvenated and reenergized, but I still was a little concerned about how I would find the time on a regular basis. I knew there had to be a compromise between the time available, and how badly I needed this break.

Searching for that balance, here's the beauty regime compromise I came up with: I promise myself just one hour, usually on the weekend, which I will spend exclusively on me. I arrange for someone to take care of the children and I make my escape alone to the bath and dressing room off our bedroom—all of which is completely off limits for the next 60 minutes. First I soak in the bath to relax. I'll usually have scented candles filling the air with my favorite perfume. Sometimes I'll put on a face pack first, or smooth on a vitamin C hair conditioner to moisturize my hair so it's being given a special treatment while I soak. After my soak I'll do my nails and toenails. If I don't spend all the time in the tub, I may putter around my dressing room with the face pack on, perhaps sorting out my dresser drawers, or organizing my cosmetics and tossing out the old tubes of mascara or the lipsticks I don't really use.

Little things like that make life so much more pleasant. Most people assume that I have all the time in the world to go out and have all this done professionally, and I might, if I didn't have children. But like you, I scrape and fight for moments I can spend alone just as earnestly as I scrape and fight to be sure I have time with my children. My first priority is to be with the children rather than to sit in a salon for two or three hours. My next priority is to take good care of myself so that when I'm with them I'm relaxed and ready for them.

If giving yourself a manicure isn't your idea of relaxation, maybe your special hour will be spent reading a favorite book and enjoying a cup of tea in a quiet room. Massage is a great treat too, especially if you can afford to have someone come to your house.

I know my shoulders and arms were really sore as the twins got heavier. In any case, I hope you'll take the time to plan out your own weekly pampering time, and then enjoy whatever it is that makes you feel most cared-for!

As you will see in your life with twins, taking care of yourself is of prime importance. It does take so much energy to care for two infants, and then to keep up with two toddlers. But I believe parents of twins are specially challenged because so many of them are no longer in their 20s—or even in their 30s. At a preschool parent meeting recently, looking around at the other mothers I was acutely aware that I was surrounded by older mothers in the room. It's no secret that I'll be 50 when the boys are in kindergarten. For the most part, that gives me a wonderful feeling because James and I are so lucky to have these boys at all, and especially lucky to have them considering our ages.

But this also gives me pause. Plenty of couples our age are sort of cruising to the finish line in terms of their families. Their children were born when they were in their 20s, and now that the

Natural Paths to Health

While conventional medicine is certainly a god-send, alternative herbal and homeopathic treatments can be a great addition. Here are some favorites Jane keeps on hand for herself and her children:

Aloe vera gel—a gentle pain reliever for sore nipples when you're breast feeding.

Calendula cream—its antiseptic qualities make it useful for treating rashes and small abrasions.

Chamomile tea or extract—soothing for upset tummies, and helpful for teething infants.

parents are in their 50s, the children are long since grown. Some of them even have young grandchildren at our age—and here we are with kindergartners! I don't ever regret having Johnny and Kris, but there have been times when I've wondered how we'll keep up with them as we get older.

James and I have talked a great deal about this issue, and here's what we've come up with. First, so much of how we live our lives begins in our minds and with how we choose to feel about ourselves and about our bodies. I really believe we can decide to feel our age or not, so quite a bit of how we feel as older parents has to do with our attitudes. At the same time, as parents we have to physically come up with the energy to run around after small children, to pick up those babies and carry two of them around here, there and everywhere. We have to be able to do the little leagues, the soccer games. It can be exhausting.

And that led James and I to the most important changes of all. When we had these babies, suddenly it was crystal clear to us that in order to do all this, we'd better become very healthy. We

Echinacea—a few drops of the tincture in water or juice helps boost the immune system.

Arnica—tiny pills to take, or a soothing cream to rub on, quiets muscle pain from a big workout, or the soreness of everyday childhood bumps and bruises.

Rescue Remedy—a natural flower essence that is remarkably effective at calming anxiety and stressful feelings—for mothers and for babies!

Each of these is available at any good health food store.

couldn't be 20 any more, but we could be extremely healthy, energetic 50-year-olds. The first thing we did was reevaluate our diet, and we made some healthy changes. On a normal day, we'll both have yogurt and fruit for breakfast, which James tops with low fat granola and I often combine with protein powder in a smoothie. Lunch is a delicious salad or Asian food we order in from a restaurant that will prepare everything without fat. And dinner is equally simple: brown rice or potatoes with some grilled vegetables and grilled fish, salad and maybe a glass of wine. I find that we actually eat quite a bit of food—lots of fruit, vegetables and whole grains—but all of them are foods that promote our health.

Both of us stay away from sweets and fats and we've found that we feel better when we do. I'm not religious about it. I know for example, that because I choose not to have those things today, it doesn't mean I'll never taste them again. It's just that I have found I can keep myself healthier and have more energy if I don't eat those things very often.

James and I also began taking a variety of supplements and herbs to be sure we were getting the vitamins and minerals we needed, and to boost our immune systems. Soon enough, your two sweet little creatures will go off to preschool and bring back their colds to share with you and all your friends! Children are amazingly adept at spreading germs you haven't encountered in the workplace. Twins also are known for infecting and re-infecting each other. While that can ultimately strengthen their immune systems, it can be a challenge to yours.

Armed with our newly revitalized healthful habits and with our positive attitudes, so far James and I have found that when we've needed energy for dealing with young twins, we've found it. We're not the 50-year-olds whose kids are off at college, facing an empty house. We're not settling down and scheduling a lot of golf to fill our days. We are however, on the golf course most weekends with our five-year-olds, teaching them the game. After golf, we'll hit a tennis ball back and forth a while. Then perhaps we'll be off for a swim with the boys.

No, we're not cruising in to the finish line. We've only just begun this marvelous journey.

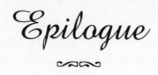

Epilogue

What can I say as a parting word to you, except that these boys have been the greatest gift in our lives, and that I know that your twins will be the same in yours. Watching my boys as they play on the grass behind our house, or kissing their chubby cheeks as I tuck them into bed, I know that any hardships or dangers I may have gone through during the pregnancy and the birth are now completely immaterial. I've only dredged them up for this book so that you can see the inner workings of twin pregnancy and birth in our lives. I hope that by sharing our experience, James and I have somehow enhanced your own.

It was not an easy road we traveled to have Kris and John, and the casual observer might ask, "Would you do it all again this way, even knowing the dangers?"

The answer is simple: Absolutely.

Would I personally go through all the ups and downs and frustrations of this pregnancy? Yes, for the obvious reason that we were given these wonderful twins as a result. But I think there's another reason that's also important. I think I appreciate these boys more than I ever would have appreciated them if they'd come easily. I don't know if everyone would say that is the right attitude to have, but I think that's how we are as humans sometimes: We blithely take the most amazing things for granted. Our bumpy road during the boys' pregnancy and birth taught us to stop taking for granted every bit of good fortune we'd been given.

The impact our twins have had on our lives and on the lives of our other children, our friends, and on our relationship is also extraordinary. It seems like they're just a couple of little magic people who have brought a sense of wonder to us all. And it's not just my twins who are this way. I talk to other families with twins, and so many feel equally blessed. We all see magic and wonder in our own double blessing, and we can't ask for more than that.

If you've already had your twins, do you look back on your pregnancy and wish you'd done some things differently? I know I do. Now that my boys are ready to start school and I've had years to reflect on this, I'm beginning to understand that many mothers feel this way, perhaps simply because none of us is perfect. I, for example, wish I'd rested more while I was pregnant. It was very hard for me—as it is for everyone—to accept the idea of bed rest, and I resisted it so much. I'd be up walking around the house and remember that I should be lying down. As soon as I'd lie down I'd remember I'd left something somewhere else, and so I'd rationalize getting up again. I do feel some remorse about that. Some days I wonder if I would have been able to change the way my pregnancy ended if I'd rested more, but Dr. Ross assures me that no one has a crystal ball in these matters. We couldn't see the future then, and of course none of us can change the past. I believe I did the best I could at the time, but sometimes I wish my best had been better.

So with the wisdom of hindsight I would urge you, if you are still pregnant, to do your best now to keep yourself and your babies healthy, so that years from now, you won't be second-guessing yourself. And if like me, you've had your babies and wish you'd done some things differently, I'd ask you to give yourself the same gentle forgiveness you'd offer your children.

When we're out with the boys now, people who don't have twins often say to us, "It must be so much work!" James loves to tell them, "No, what I do all day is a lot of work. Whatever I do with Kris and Johnny is a lot of joy! Even when they're screaming or crying—all that's temporary. It changes in an eye blink anyway—and you're left with the joy."

He likes to remind those who think that having twins is too much work—and I like to remind myself—that when you ask for one and you're given two, you've received a gift that's beyond generous. James and I believe that when one is lucky enough to receive such a gift, there is nothing better to do than to feel immense gratitude, and then to somehow share that blessing with other families.

And we wish the same for you and your twins.

Index

Page numbers in *italics* indicate illustrations.